Schizophrenia:
Challenging the

Edited by

Colm McDonald
Wellcome Trust Research Training Fellow
Division of Psychological Medicine
Institute of Psychiatry
London
UK

Katja Schulze
Research Psychologist
Division of Psychological Medicine
Institute of Psychiatry
London
UK

Robin M Murray
Professor of Psychiatry
Division of Psychological Medicine
Institute of Psychiatry
London
UK

Pádraig Wright
Honorary Senior Lecturer
Division of Psychological Medicine
Institute of Psychiatry
London
UK

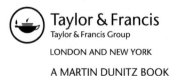

Taylor & Francis
Taylor & Francis Group

LONDON AND NEW YORK

A MARTIN DUNITZ BOOK

European Foundation for Psychiatry
at The Maudsley

© 2004 Taylor & Francis, an imprint of the Taylor & Francis Group

First published in the United Kingdom in 2004
by Taylor & Francis, an imprint of the Taylor & Francis Group, 11 New Fetter Lane,
London EC4P 4EE

Tel.:   +44 (0) 20 7583 9855
Fax.:   +44 (0) 20 7842 2298
E-mail: info@dunitz.co.uk
Website: http://www.dunitz.co.uk

Although every effort has been made to ensure that all owners of copyright material have been acknowledged in this publication, we would be glad to acknowledge in sub-sequent reprints or editions any omissions brought to our attention.

Although every effort has been made to ensure that drug doses and other information are presented accurately in this publication, the ultimate responsibility rests with the prescribing physician. Neither the publishers nor the authors can be held responsible for errors or for any consequences arising from the use of information contained herein. For detailed prescribing information or instructions on the use of any product or procedure discussed herein, please consult the prescribing information or instruc-tional material issued by the manufacturer.

A CIP record for this book is available from the British Library.
Library of Congress Cataloging-in-Publication Data
Data available on application

ISBN 1 84184 378 4

Cover artwork by Peter Rowbotham

Composition by Wearset Ltd, Boldon, Tyne and Wear, UK

Printed and bound in Italy by Printer Trento

Contents

Section III: Epidemiology: Anyone can find an environmental risk factor

**Section IV: The prodrome and early intervention: More than
a marketing ploy?**

**Section V: Psychopharmacology and psychology:
Do the two worlds ever meet?**

Foreword

The late Bob Kendall once described schizophrenia as 'the heartland of psychiatry'. I think by this he meant that the disorder is not just central to the practice of psychiatry but that, by its nature, tackling schizophrenia presents a core intellectual challenge that is almost bound to both fascinate and intrigue the clinician. Understanding schizophrenia, discovering its causes and devising more effective therapies also form territories that every researcher would aspire to conquer. At the same time schizophrenia has long been a chief focus of debate and disagreement that somehow has never been the case concerning, for example, mood disorders.

Although it is no longer fashionable, as it once was, to propose that schizophrenia is a 'myth' or that it is in some way a 'sane response to an insane world', it is still not uncommon to hear some senior clinical psychologists (and an occasional psychiatrist) suggest that the diagnosis should be abandoned altogether. This is at a time when, whatever its merits and demerits, the movement towards 'care in the community' has ensured that schizophrenia and those who suffer from the disorder are more visible to the general public and are in receipt of more media attention than has been the case since Bleuler first coined the term. We are also in a period where, despite moans about inadequate clinical research funding by those of us who are engaged in it, there is almost certainly more scientific research on schizophrenia currently being conducted and more publication of research papers than has ever been the case.

This book is therefore timely in several respects. In covering in its seven themes of brain imaging, genetics, environmental risk factors, early interventions, animal and pharmacological models, cognitive therapies and diagnostic issues, it addresses most of the big questions that schizophrenia researchers and clinicians are forced to grapple with. Moreover, the editors have requested their authors to adopt a deliberately challenging and provocative approach so that the result is not just another standard text but instead is a lively and critical account that the reader will find both stimulating and demanding. We are at a stage of real technical advances. For example, new imaging methods enable the production of astounding pictures of the brain's structure and how it functions. We are also, at last, beginning to see tangible results in the search for the molecular genetic basis of schizophrenia. However in this volume achievements such as these are not simply taken for granted as representing 'progress'; their value is scrutinized with a healthy degree of scepticism. Similarly, currently fashionable treatment approaches such as early intervention with medication and the use of various cognitive approaches that are employed in talking treatments are given a fair but critical hearing.

Although the book follows on from the first meeting of the European Foundation for Psychiatry at the Maudsley, its approach is not I think parochial to this, the smallest and most densely populated continent. Rather it should represent a thoroughly worthwhile read in whatever corner of the globe its reader sits.

Peter McGuffin
Director, MRC, Social, Genetic
and Developmental Psychiatry Centre
Institute of Psychiatry
King's College London

Preface

Despite enormous efforts and some significant therapeutic advances, schizo-phrenia remains the most chronic and disabling of the major mental illnesses. The disorder is a huge burden, not only because of the direct suffering of patients and their relatives, but also through the wider economic costs to society at large. Before we can understand the causes of schizophrenia and optimize its management, it is vital to critically examine the (often dubious) evidence supporting established opinions about this disorder. To this end, over 250 delegates from 13 countries across Europe attended the inaugural meeting of the European Foundation for Psychiatry at the Maudsley, held at the Institute of Psychiatry in London. The purpose of this conference was to question many of the dogmas about the illness, and explore new and more pro-ductive ways of thinking about it. This volume arises from that conference.

Schizophrenia: Challenging the Orthodox comprises seven thematic sections. The first centres on neuroimaging. The early CT studies rescued the biological foundations of schizophrenia and re-established it, for some, as a 'brain' disease. Since that time advances in neuroimaging have allowed the application of ever improving techniques to the illness, including high resolution structural MRI to better delineate subtle volumetric brain changes and functional imaging to examine regional brain dysfunction. Newer techniques such as diffusion tensor imaging examine the disturbances of white matter connections between critical nodes throughout the brain. The orthodox view is that these new techniques have greatly furthered our understanding of both the impaired cognitive function and characteristic symptoms of the syndrome; however, some sceptics dismiss neuroimaging as expensive but irrelevant 'medical photography' which has provided no practical help to patients.

Research into the genetics of schizophrenia is examined in the second section. Despite huge research effort, progress in the search for susceptibility genes has been painstakingly slow, with numerous false dawns over the last two decades. Indeed, some would say that the only area of human endeavour to produce so many unsubstantiated claims has been the search for alien spacecraft! However, the last couple of years have seen the first replicable results with new evidence supporting *neuregulin 1* as the first true susceptibility gene for schizophrenia and with several other promising genes emerging. An alternative view is that more immediate benefit will come from examining how variation in the genes determining neurochemical systems and enzymes responsible for drug metabolism impact upon the individual patient's response to antipsychotic medication.

The third section changes tack to examine the numerous putative non-genetic risk factors for schizophrenia and how they are identified using the powerful tools of epidemiology. Evidence is presented to argue that a range of social and physical environmental risk factors underlie schizophrenia including birth hypoxia, urban life, ethnicity, early stress, smoking, and abuse of drugs such as cannabis and methamphetamines. However, it seems unlikely that everybody's favourite risk factor will turn out to be true – the problem is how to tell the difference between real and imaginary causal risk factors. Also in this section, the boundaries of the schizophrenic syndrome are examined in the light of how social risk factors predispose to lesser psychotic-like symptoms on a dimension which extends to normality. Attention is also paid to understanding the heavy emotional impact of psychosis on the individual.

The idea that intervention at the earliest possible opportunity, even before the onset of frank psychosis, might improve outcome for patients, has been the focus of intense research in recent years and has attracted proponents with evangelical zeal. This section includes some of the more enthusiastic proponents and also examines some of the conceptual, practical and research design issues surrounding this area. On the one hand, data are described which demonstrate that the prediction of transition to psychosis from prodromal symptoms and the reduction of the duration of untreated psychosis are achievable goals. On the other hand, Anthony David bravely argues that the resources necessary to implement early detection and treatment programs would be better spent on developing the therapeutic strategies that we already know improve outcome in those suffering more, e.g. increasing compliance in those already ill.

The fifth section asks whether evidence from the widely varying research techniques of psychopharmacology, psychology, and animal models can be integrated to further our understanding of the neurochemical dysfunction which underlies the experience of psychosis, and centres particularly on dysregulation of the dopamine system.

Until the 1990s it was almost impossible to get psychologists to express any interest in the treatment of schizophrenia. This situation has now greatly changed in Europe but not yet in North America where most psychiatrists maintain that it is impossible to change beliefs by psychological means – perhaps the obstinacy with which they themselves hold to this view is demonstration enough of how difficult it is to change beliefs! Perhaps some may be convinced by the sixth section which examines cognitive models of psychotic symptoms and how the latter can be manipulated by, for example, cognitive behavioural therapy to improve symptoms and even delay transition to psychosis, or cognitive remediation therapy to ameliorate cognitive deficit.

Many psychotic patients receive different diagnoses throughout their careers, veering from a diagnosis of schizophrenia in one episode to affective psychosis in the next (and then back again!). In the final section, the traditional dichotomy between schizophrenia and manic depression is examined in the light of recent studies investigating genetics, structural and functional neuroimaging, and premorbid deficits in the two disorders. These techniques have identified distinct but also overlapping risk factors and abnormalities, which probably contribute to the blurred clinical separation of these psychoses. Thus, it seems that while Kraepelin was not wholly right, neither was he entirely wrong.

The European Foundation for Psychiatry at the Maudsley (EFPM) is an independent body aiming to provide up-to-date knowledge to Europe's foremost clinical and academic professionals in mental health. Eli Lilly and Company provided an educational grant for the meeting but, as the reader will see from the contents of the book, there were no promotional or non-promotional talks.

We hope that *Schizophrenia: Challenging the Orthodox* will ensure that the dialogue initiated by the inaugural EFPM meeting is available to as wide an audience as possible. It will be of interest to academics within psychiatry, psychology and neuroscience as well as mental health professionals interested in schizophrenia research. The expert contributions capture the considerable progress that has been made in our understanding of this devastating disorder in recent years.

The editors are very grateful to all the contributors for their manuscripts and hope that the reader will also be stimulated and challenged by the dialectical approach that this book encompasses.

Colm McDonald
Katja Schulze
Robin M Murray
Pádraig Wright

Contributors

Maria J Arranz, *Clinical Neuropharmacology, Division of Psychological Medicine, Institute of Psychiatry, De Crespigny Park, Denmark Hill, London SE5 8AF, UK*

Louise Arseneault, *Social, Genetic and Developmental Psychiatry Research Centre, Division of Psychological Medicine, Institute of Psychiatry, De Crespigny Park, Denmark Hill, London SE5 8AF, UK*

Max Birchwood, *Director, Birmingham Early Intervention Service, Birmingham and Solihull Mental Health Trust, Professor of Mental Health, Department of Psychology, University of Birmingham, Edgbaston, Birmingham B15 2TT, UK*

Elvira Bramon, *Wellcome Trust Fellow, Division of Psychological Medicine, Institute of Psychiatry, Kings College London, De Crespigny Park, Denmark Hill, London SE5 8AF, UK*

Jon Brynjolfsson, *Consultant Psychiatrist, Saudarkrokur, Iceland*

Mary Cannon, *Senior Lecturer, Department of Psychiatry Royal College of Surgeons in Ireland; and Division of Psychological Medicine, Institute of Psychiatry, De Crespigny Park, Denmark Hill, London SE5 8AF, UK*

Chih-Ken Chen, *Division of Psychological Medicine, Institute of Psychiatry, De Crespigny Park, Denmark Hill, London SE5 8AF, UK*

Audrey Cougnard, *Department of Psychiatry and IFR of Public Health, Université Victor Segalen, Bordeaux, France*

Anthony S David, *Honorary Consultant Psychiatrist, South London and Maudsley NHS Trust; Professor of Cognitive Neuropsychiatry, Section of Neuropsychiatry, Institute of Psychiatry, De Crespigny Park, Denmark Hill, London SE5 8AF, UK*

Kimberlie Dean, *Division of Psychological Medicine, Institute of Psychiatry, De Crespigny Park, Denmark Hill, London SE5 8AF, UK*

Thomas Dierks, *Head, Department of Psychiatric Neurophysiology, University Hospital of Clinical Psychiatry, Bern, Bollingenstrasse 111, CH-3000 Bern 60, Switzerland*

Cyril D'Souza, *Associate Professor of Psychiatry, Yale University School of Medicine, Psychiatry Service 116 A, VA Connecticut Health Care System, 950 Campbell Avenue, West Haven, CT 06516, USA*

Chris D Frith, *Wellcome Principal Research Fellow, Wellcome Department of Imaging Neuroscience, Institute of Neurology, 12 Queen Square, London, WC1N 3BG, UK*

Anton Grech, *Division of Psychological Medicine, Institute of Psychiatry, De Crespigny Park, Denmark Hill, London SE5 8AF, UK*

Vala G Gudnadottir, *Reseach Scientist, deCODE genetics, Sturlugata 8, 101 Reykjavík, Iceland*

Elsa Gudmundsdottir, *Consultant Psychiatrist, Department of Psychiatry, Akureyri Hospital, Iceland*

Jeffrey R Gulcher, *Scientific Director, deCODE genetics, Sturlugata 8, 101 Reykjavík, Iceland*

Steinunn Gunnarsdottir, *Research Scientist, deCODE genetics, Sturlugata 8, 101 Reykjavík, Iceland*

Anthony A Grace, *Professor of Neuroscience, Psychiatry and Psychology, Department of Neuroscience, University of Pittsburgh, 458 Crawford Hall, Pittsburgh, PA 15260, USA*

Hronn Hardardottir, *Research Nurse, Division of Psychiatry, Landspitali University Hospital Hringbraut, Reykjavík, Iceland*

Omar Hjaltason, *Consultant Psychiatrist, Division of Psychiatry, Landspitali University Hospital, Hringbraut, Reykjavík, Iceland*

Daniela Hubl, *Research Physician, Department of Psychiatric Neurophysiology, University Hospital of Clinical Psychiatry, Bollingenstrasse 111, CH-3000 Bern 60, Switzerland*

Andres Ingason, *Research Scientist, deCODE genetics, Sturlugata 8, 101 Reykjavík, Iceland*

Brynjolfur Ingvarsson, *Consultant Psychiatrist, Department of Psychiatry, Akureyri Hospital, Iceland*

Omar Ivarsson, *Consultant Psychiatrist, Division of Psychiatry, Landspitali University Hospital, Hringbraut, Reykjavík, Iceland*

Helgi Jonsson, *Consultant Psychiatrist, Division of Psychiatry, Landspitali University Hospital, Hringbraut, Reykjavík, Iceland*

Shitij Kapur, *Canada Research Chair in Schizophrenia and Therapeutic Neuroscience, Professor of Psychiatry, Centre for Addiction and Mental Health, University of Toronto, 33 Russell Street, Toronto, M5S 2S1, Canada*

Robert W Kerwin, *Professor of Clinical Neuropharmacology, Division of Psychological Medicine, Institute of Psychiatry, De Crespigny Park, Denmark Hill, London SE5 8AF, UK*

Lydia Krabbendam, *Lecturer, Department of Psychiatry and Neuropsychology, Institute of Brain and Behaviour, Maastricht University, 6200 MD Maastricht, The Netherlands*

Tor K Larsen, *Associate Professor of Psychiatry, Helse Stavanger HF, Psychiatric Clinic, Armauer Hansensv. 20, PO Box 8100, N-4068 Stavanger, Norway*

Glyn Lewis, *Professor of Psychiatric Epidemiology, University of Bristol, Cotham House, Cotham Hill, Bristol BS6 6JL, UK*

Shôn Lewis, *Professor, School of Psychiatry and Behavioural Sciences, University of Manchester, Education and Research Centre, Wythenshawe Hospital, Manchester M23 9LT, UK*

David C Mamo, *Research Fellow and Psychiatrist, PET Centre, Schizophrenia and Continuing Care Program, Centre for Addiction and Mental Health, Department of Psychiatry, University of Toronto, 250 College Street, Toronto, M5T 1R8, Canada*

Dalu Mancama, *Research Fellow, Clinical Neuropharmacology, Division of Psychological Medicine, Institute of Psychiatry, De Crespigny Park, Denmark Hill, London SE5 8AF, UK*

Colm McDonald, *Wellcome Trust Research Training Fellow, Division of Psychological Medicine, Institute of Psychiatry, De Crespigny Park, Denmark Hill, London SE5 8AF, UK*

Philip K McGuire, *Professor, Section of Neuroimaging, Institute of Psychiatry, De Crespigny Park, Denmark Hill, London SE5 8AF, UK*

Robin M Murray, *Professor of Psychiatry, Division of Psychological Medicine, Institute of Psychiatry, De Crespigny Park, Denmark Hill, London SE5 8AF, UK*

Nadine Norton, *Post-doctoral Research Scientist, Department of Psychological Medicine, Henry Wellcome Building, University of Wales College of Medicine, Heath Park, Cardiff CF14 4XN, UK*

Michael J Owen, *Professor, Neuropsychiatric Genetics Unit, Head, Department of Psychological Medicine, Henry Wellcome Building, University of Wales College of Medicine, Heath Park, Cardiff CF14 4XN, UK*

Hannes Petursson, *Professor of Psychiatry, Division of Psychiatry, Landspitali University Hospital, Hringbraut, 101 Reykjavík, Iceland*

Mary L Phillips, *Professor of Neuroscience and Emotion in Psychiatry, Head of Section of Neuroscience and Emotion, Honorary Consultant Psychiatrist, Division of Psychological Medicine, Institute of Psychiatry and GKT School of Medicine, De Crespigny Park, Denmark Hill, London SE5 8AF, UK*

Katja Schulze, *Research Psychologist, Division of Psychological Medicine, Institute of Psychiatry, De Crespigny Park, Denmark Hill, London SE5 8AF, UK*

Frauke Schultze-Lutter, *Early recognition and Intervention Centre for Mental Crisis, FETZ, Department of Psychiatry and Psychotherapy, University of Cologne, Joseph-Stelzmann-Str. 9, 50924 Cologne, Germany*

Pak Sham, *Professor of Psychiatric and Statistical Genetics, Social Genetic and Development Psychiatry Research Group, Institute of Psychiatry, Kings College London, De Crespigny Park, Denmark Hill, London SE5 8AF, UK*

Sigmundur Sigfusson, *Consultant Psychiatrist, Department of Psychiatry, Akureyri Hospital, Iceland*

Thordur Sigmundsson, *Consultant Psychiatrist, Division of Psychiatry, Landspitali University Hospital, Hringbraut, 101 Reykjavík, Iceland*

Engilbert Sigurdsson, *Docent and Consultant Psychiatrist, Division of Psychiatry, Landspitali University Hospital, Hringbraut, 101 Reykjavík, Iceland*

Hreinn Stefansson, *Head of CNS Division, deCODE genetics, Sturlugata 8, 101 Reykjavík, Iceland*

Kari Stefansson, *Chief Executive Officer, deCODE genetics, Sturlugata 8, 101 Reykjavík, Iceland*

Valgerdur Steinthorsdottir, *Research Scientist, deCODE genetics, Sturlugata 8, 101 Reykjavík, Iceland*

Jim van Os, *Department of Psychiatry and Neuropsychology, Institute of Brain and Behaviour, Maastricht University, 6200 MD Maastricht, The Netherlands*

Hélène Verdoux, *Professor of Adult Psychiatry, Department of Psychiatry, Université Victor Segalen Bordeaux 2, Hôpital Charles Perrens, 121 Rue de la Béchade, 33076 Bordeaux Cedex, France*

Pádraig Wright, *Honorary Senior Lecturer, Division of Psychological Medicine, Institute of Psychiatry, De Crespigny Park, London, SE5 8AF, UK*

Til Wykes, *Professor and Head of the Centre for Recovery in Severe Psychosis, Department of Psychology, Institute of Psychiatry, De Crespigny Park, London SE5 8AF, UK*

Stan Zammit, *Lecturer, Department of Psychological Medicine, University of Wales College of Medicine, Cardiff, Wales, UK*

Jolanta Zanelli, *Division of Psychological Medicine, Institute of Psychiatry, De Crespigny Park, Denmark Hill, London SE5 8AF, UK*

chapter 1

Brain abnormalities in schizophrenia and in those at risk of it

Philip McGuire

While it is clear that schizophrenia is associated with structural and functional abnormalities of the brain, the extent to which these are related to a vulnerability to schizophrenia as opposed to the presence of the disorder itself is less certain. This issue can be addressed through comparison of people at increased risk of schizophrenia (but who are not psychotic) and patients with the disorder.

One group at increased risk that has been widely studied comprises the relatives of people with schizophrenia, particularly first degree relatives. There have several studies that have compared this group with their relatives who have schizophrenia and with healthy controls. In general, in terms of neuroanatomical abnormalities, the relatives of patients lie between patients and healthy volunteers, although this varies to some extent with the structure in question. For example, if one looks at ventricular volume, then the ventriculomegaly seen in schizophrenia is also evident in those at risk of schizophrenia, but to a lesser degree.[1] Similarly, relatives appear to have medial temporal volumes which are smaller than in controls but larger than in patients with schizophrenia.[2]

However, in studies of the relatives of patients it is difficult to quantify the magnitude of risk in an individual. This is less of an issue if familial risk is examined in twins, particularly those who are genetically identical but are discordant for schizophrenia. Again there have been a number of neuroimaging studies in this area. Baare et al found that in genetically identical twin pairs, schizophrenia was associated with a reduction in total cortical volume and enlarged ventricles.[3] However, there also seemed to be an effect of risk on intracranial volume, so both the disorder and the degree of genetic risk appeared to have neural correlates. In another recent study in twins, Cannon et al reported that schizophrenia was associated with less grey matter in a number of regions, particularly the lateral prefrontal, parietal and temporal cortex.[4] Genetic vulnerability to schizophrenia across monozygotic (MZ) and dizygotic (DZ) twins was associated with volume reductions in a different set of areas, although these overlapped with those associated with the presence of schizophrenia, particularly in the lateral prefrontal cortex. Thus, in some areas, cortical volume appeared to depend on both the individual's genetic risk and whether they were affected by the disorder.

The effect of familial risk of schizophrenia has been less widely studied with functional than structural neuroimaging. However, while the functional abnormalities associated with schizophrenia may be less robust than volumetric changes, functional imaging is likely to be more sensitive to subtle changes in the brain. Recent research on twins at the Institute of Psychiatry, London, has used functional magnetic resonance imaging (MRI) to this end, in conjunction with a verbal self-monitoring paradigm which is associated with both behavioural and functional abnormalities in patients with schizophrenia.[5,6] Normally when we speak we hear our own voice and we know what it is going to sound like. Altering the pitch of the speech such that the subject's voice sounds slightly different to that expected engages verbal self-monitoring, which is thought to be one of the key cognitive processes impaired in schizophrenia.[7] Picchioni et al scanned MZ twins who were discordant for schizophrenia and healthy MZ twins while they carried out this task.[8] The preliminary data indicate that twins with schizophrenia showed a marked reduction in prefrontal and temporal cortical activation relative to healthy twins, while the non-psychotic co-twins of the patients showed a level of temporal activation that was intermediate between that in the other two groups (Figure 1.1). So in this sample it appears that both the vulnerability to schizophrenia and the disorder affected brain function in these areas.

All the above studies were cross-sectional, and when comparing different groups of subjects, it is difficult to exclude the possibility that the findings were related to a between-group difference in a variable other than the parameter of interest. This potential confound can be overcome in a prospective design if a subject is studied when vulnerable to schizophrenia and then again when they subsequently develop the disorder. This approach has been used to study the relatives of patients with schizophrenia in the Edinburgh

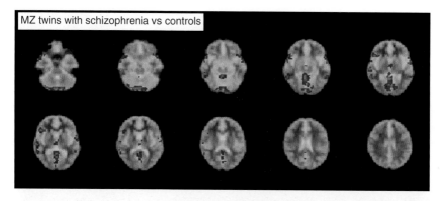

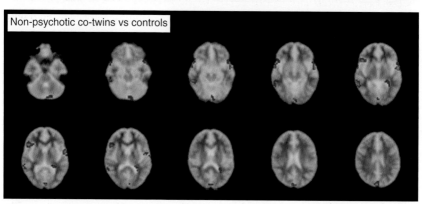

Figure 1.1 Brain activation during a verbal self-monitoring task in monozygotic (MZ) twins discordant for schizophrenia. Non-psychotic co-twins of patients with schizophrenia showed reduced activation compared to healthy controls in qualitatively similar areas to those showing reduced activation in their psychotic co-twins. However, functional abnormalities were more extensive in the twins with schizophrenia than their co-twins.[8]

High Risk study, but entails the scanning and follow up of large numbers of subjects, as the proportion of high risk subjects who go on to develop psychosis is relatively small. A different vulnerable group with a higher risk of transition to psychosis are people who have 'prodromal' symptoms, or an 'at risk mental state'. If followed up for 12 months, up to 40% may develop psychosis within this period.[9] Pantelis et al used MRI to scan a group of people with prodromal symptoms and then followed them up for 12 months.[10] Comparison of the baseline MRI data from subjects who later developed psychosis with those who did not revealed that the former group showed less grey matter volume in the inferior frontal and cingulate cortex than the latter at the prodromal stage, despite the subgroups being clinically similar. This suggests that within this high risk group, those destined to develop

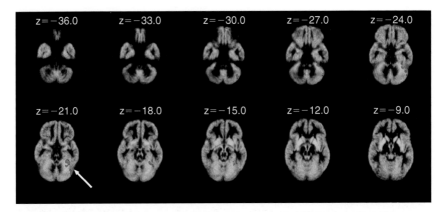

Figure 1.2 *Evidence of progressive changes associated with the transition from the 'at risk mental state' to psychosis. A longitudinal reduction in volume was particularly evident in the left medial temporal lobe (arrow). (Reproduced from Pantelis C et al[10] with permission.)*

psychosis showed volumetric reductions compared to those who were not. The second component of this study involved repeating the MRI scans at 12 months follow up. In the subgroup who had become psychotic, there was a reduction in the volume of the left medial temporal cortex between the baseline and follow up scans, a change that was not evident in subjects who did not become psychotic (Figure 1.2). These data suggest that the structure of the brain in people with an 'at-risk mental state' already differs from that in controls, and that further volumetric differences emerge with the onset of psychosis.

Overall, the studies that have been discussed indicate that some of the abnormalities that are associated with schizophrenia are also evident in people at high risk of developing the disorder, whether this be through a genetic vulnerability or via the presence of prodromal symptoms. However, the magnitude of these abnormalities may be greater in patients with the disorder than those at risk, and there may also be abnormalities that are particularly associated with the presence of psychosis. This would be consistent with the pattern of clinical features and neuropsychological impairments in patients, at-risk individuals and controls. Thus, in general, in those at increased risk of schizophrenia the severity of psychiatric symptoms and cognitive deficits is roughly intermediate between that in healthy individuals and patients with the disorder.

References

1. Sharma T, Lancaster E, Sigmundsson T et al, Lack of normal pattern of cerebral asymmetry in familial schizophrenic patients and their relatives – the Maudsley Family Study. *Schizophr Res* 1999; **40**:111–120.
2. Lawrie SM, Whalley H, Kestelman JN et al, Magnetic resonance imaging of brain in people at high risk of developing schizophrenia. *Lancet* 1999; **353**:30–33.
3. Baare W, van Oel C, Hulshoff H et al, Volumes of brain structures in twins discordant for schizophrenia. *Arch Gen Psychiatry* 2001; **58**:33–40.
4. Cannon T, Thompson P, van Erp T et al, A probabilistic atlas of cortical gray matter changes in monozygotic twins discordant for schizophrenia. *Neuroimage* 2001; **13**:S1034.
5. Johns L, McGuire PK, Verbal self-monitoring and auditory hallucinations in schizophrenia. *Lancet* 1999; **353**:469–470.
6. Fu C, McGuire PK, Verbal self-monitoring. In: Kircher T, David A, eds, *The Self in Neuroscience and Psychiatry*, 425–435, Cambridge: Cambridge University Press.
7. Frith CD, Done DJ, Towards a neuropsychology of schizophrenia. *Br J Psychiatry* 1987; **153**:437–443.
8. Picchioni MM, Chitnis XA, Fu CHY et al, Functional imaging of verbal self monitoring in monozygotic twins discordant for schizophrenia. *Am J Med Genet* 2002; **114**:866.
9. Yung AR, Phillips LJ, McGorry PD et al, Prediction of psychosis. A step towards indicated prevention of schizophrenia. *Br J Psychiatry Suppl* 1998; **172**: 14–20.
10. Pantelis C, Velakoulis D, McGorry P et al, Neuroanatomical abnormalities in people who develop psychosis. *Lancet* 2003; **361**:281–288.

chapter 2

Visualizing the cerebral alterations that underlie auditory hallucinations in schizophrenia

Daniela Hubl and Thomas Dierks

Auditory hallucinations, one of the most common symptoms in schizophrenia, have eluded a definitive explanation since antiquity. They have been discussed in nearly every conceivable context, from a very private experience to an abnormal brain function in the setting of schizophrenia. Auditory hallucinations occur frequently in hospitalized psychiatric patients and are often torturous because of their highly emotional and personal content. In addition, patients report that they perceive the acoustic quality of auditory hallucinations to be like – and often the same as – real, spoken words. In many cases, patients can point to the direction from where they perceive the voices. One challenge for modern brain research in schizophrenia is as follows: What makes these voices sound so real?

Early observations

In the early nineteenth century, the concept of a brain-based origin of hallucinations, which contradicted the traditional view of possession, was formulated. Although auditory hallucinations occur with a lifetime prevalence of 10–15% in persons without neuropsychiatric disease, they are most common in patients with schizophrenia, with an average prevalence of 60%.[1] Recent concepts of auditory hallucinations therefore have been based on results primarily from investigations of patients with schizophrenia. Research support for abnormalities of the left temporal lobe, including the auditory cortices, being associated with auditory hallucinations was provided from early neuropathological studies.[2] Recently, in vivo volumetric magnetic resonance imaging (MRI) studies have further supported these earlier findings, describing correlations between the volume of the left superior temporal gyrus and the severity of auditory hallucinations.[3] The examination of the psychopathology of auditory hallucinations and in vivo structural MRI studies, however, do not allow direct observation of the rapidly fluctuating symptoms of this condition. To investigate the functional dynamics of auditory hallucinations, methods with considerable temporal and spatial resolution are needed. Another difficulty in investigating patients who have schizophrenia with auditory hallucinations is that most of these patients are in an acute stage of their psychosis. Other symptoms of acute schizophrenia, such as a lack of concentration and attention, suspiciousness, and cognitive dysfunction, can make it difficult to investigate auditory hallucinations. Nevertheless, for a better understanding of the complex functional and pathophysiological underpinnings of auditory hallucinations the application of functional imaging methods is needed.

Methodological overview

With the improvements in functional imaging and electrophysiological techniques, it has become possible to investigate the brain in vivo during dynamic processes such as auditory hallucinations. In addition to improved imaging techniques, methodological advances over the past decade have refined the investigation of auditory hallucinations. Single-photon emission computed tomography (SPECT) and positron emission tomography (PET) are imaging techniques that allow metabolic and functional information about the brain tissue to be obtained in vivo. However, these methods with a resolution in the subcentimetre scale lack the higher spatial resolution of MRI or computed tomography which are reaching into the millimetre scale. Furthermore, the temporal resolution is commonly in the scale of minutes to hours (depending on the tracer). In addition, these methods are indirectly invasive, in that intravenous radioactive markers must be applied to map the metabolic alterations.

The development of the newer method of functional MRI (fMRI) is a significant improvement compared to previous imaging techniques.[4] fMRI is non-invasive, has a spatial resolution in the range of millimetres, and has a temporal resolution in the range of seconds, or less. This technique uses the different magnetic features of oxygenated and deoxygenated haemoglobin as a contrast agent, and thus allows the indirect investigation of neuronal activity by measuring vascular effects. These effects can be measured by using special MRI sequences, the so-called 'blood oxygen level-dependent' (BOLD) signal-sensitive sequences.

Another new MRI technique, which has begun to enter standard MRI protocols, is magnetic resonance diffusion tensor imaging (MR-DTI or DTI).[5] DTI allows non-invasive, in vivo investigations of white matter microstructure. DTI is based on MR signals that are sensitized to the movement of water. If there are no oriented diffusion barriers, as in cerebrospinal fluid, water diffusion occurs isotropically. In cerebral white matter, the nerve fibres, with their myelin sheaths and cell membranes, present boundaries, and diffusion will occur preferentially along the fibres. This directed diffusion characteristic is called anisotropy. Most commonly the fractional anisotropy (FA) is computed, which is a scalar measure, ranging between 0 and 1, in which higher values indicate greater directionality – thus a more coherent orientation of fibres – and lower values indicate lower white matter integrity or disruption of the microstructure.

Applications

The earliest functional imaging studies of auditory hallucinations, in the late 1980s, used SPECT and PET, because these were the only techniques available at the time. Most protocols used a group of patients with auditory hallucinations and compared them with patients without hallucinations who had schizophrenia or with healthy controls. More advanced protocols reported on the same group of patients, using the time point when they perceived their auditory hallucinations and a later time point when the auditory hallucinations had disappeared. This procedure had the following drawback: often, the patient's psychopharmacological medication had changed and, in some cases, the second measurement could not be done until months later. Despite these shortcomings, the studies resulted in findings of an association of auditory hallucinations and activation of the left temporal lobe, where the auditory cortices are located. Further activation of the frontal language regions, basal ganglia and thalamus, hippocampal region, and anterior cingulate gyri (most of them bilateral) has been described (for a review see reference 6).

With the development of refined imaging protocols, the investigation of the dynamic processes in auditory hallucinations has improved. The first PET study investigating patients as their own controls by measuring their cerebral blood flow during hallucinating and quiescent periods showed an increased activation when auditory hallucinations occurred in the subcortical nuclei (thalamic and striatal) and parts of the limbic system (i.e. hippocampus, parahippocampus, cingulate gyrus).[7] The cortical activations were mainly distributed to the temporoparietal cortex. The activation of deep brain nuclei was believed to generate or modulate the auditory hallucinations, and the sensory cortical region may have affected the perceptual content. Although state and trait investigations pointed to an involvement of the language and auditory system in auditory hallucinations, clear evidence for an activation of the primary auditory cortex (PAC) was missing. Significantly, an activation of the PAC (Heschl's gyrus) could provide an explanation for the reason why patients perceive the auditory hallucinations as real as spoken speech, because this activation would be comparable to that evoked via external acoustic stimuli. Therefore, we wanted to investigate whether the PAC is activated during auditory hallucinations.

We used fMRI as a high-resolution technique and a protocol that was customized on the dynamic processes of auditory hallucinations – namely, their fluctuations (onset and termination of auditory hallucinations).[8] During one fMRI session, patients were scanned while they were perceiving auditory hallucinations and when the auditory hallucinations stopped. The subjects were asked to indicate by pressing a button the onset and the end of their auditory hallucinations. Because high cognitive performance is needed in patients with schizophrenia during their acute state of hallucinations, only eight patients could be investigated. Correlation of the BOLD signal time course with the subjective experience of auditory hallucination resulted in a unilateral activation of Heschl's gyrus (Figure 2.1) in each of the subjects. This supports the subjective report of the patients that they heard real voices due to an objective verifiable activation of the auditory system. We found that the activation of the PAC was always in the dominant hemisphere. In addition, we found significant increases of the BOLD signal in the hippocampus, amygdala, Broca's area, and the primary motor cortex (Figure 2.2A).

Auditory hallucinations can be described by many characteristics, including their physical features, content, relation to personal memories and affective impact. It would be beneficial to know whether the activation in the different brain regions, each representing aspects of the different features, follows a certain activation order. To investigate this, we measured, in

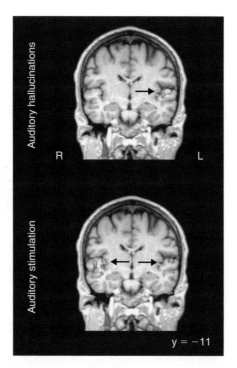

Figure 2.1 *Upper figure: During auditory hallucinations activation of the primary auditory cortex (PAC; black arrow) could be observed in functional magnetic resonance imaging. Lower figure: To localize the PAC and verify the results an acoustic activation paradigm was used. The activations are presented superimposed on two coronal anatomical slices. The localization of the activations during auditory hallucinations and the PAC coincide.*

a detailed analysis of one patient, the peak latency of the BOLD signal for each of the activated regions, relative to the earliest BOLD maximum (Figure 2.2B). This measurement resulted in a sequential activation of the hippocampus (1) and nearly simultaneous activation of the Broca's area (2). The activation of the amygdala (3) and PAC (4) followed somewhat later. Finally, the primary motor cortex (5) was activated. We interpreted this sequence of pathological activation in the following way: memories come up (1), nearly simultaneously the motor speech area (2) is activated. This seems to be related to an erroneous functional connection between subjective memories and language system. Broca's area is a motor speech area and thus is relevant for the generation of inner speech, one mechanism considered to be important for the generation of auditory hallucinations. Somewhat later, the activation of the amygdala (3) contributes to the emotional coloration of the

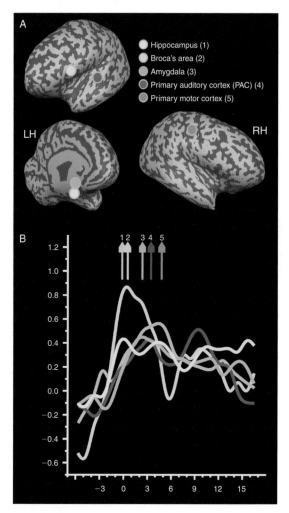

Figure 2.2 *(A) Additionally to the primary auditory cortex (PAC) activation, significant blood oxygen level-dependent (BOLD) signal increases were observed in hippocampus, Broca's area, amygdala, and primary motor cortex. The location of these five regions is schematically presented on an inflated cortical surface. (B) Analysis of the BOLD signal time course pointed to a sequential activation of hippocampus, Broca's area, amygdala, PAC, and primary motor cortex. The colour codes in (A) and (B) correspond to each other.*

auditory hallucinations, and the activation of PAC (4) makes this mixture of memory, inner speech and emotional content heard. Finally, the patient realizes that the auditory hallucination has begun and presses the button to indicate the beginning of the hallucination. These results support not only the hypothesis that auditory hallucinations are related to inner speech but also provide evidence that they are perceived as real, spoken speech via activation of the PAC.

Another activation study, using acoustic stimulation, described a lack of activation of the auditory regions in hallucinating patients with schizophrenia compared with patients without auditory hallucinations.[9] This finding points to a reduced responsivity in the PAC during auditory hallucinations and supports indirectly our finding of a pathological activation of PAC. A concept of auditory hallucinations and external stimuli competing for common neurophysiological resources in the auditory system can be hypothesized.

Present hypothesis of generation and origin of auditory hallucinations

Imaging studies of the past decade in patients with auditory hallucinations have shown a dysfunction in language-related cerebral regions and aberrant activation of the primary and higher order auditory and association cortex, mainly located in the frontal and temporal lobes, primarily in the left hemisphere of the brain. From these findings, the present hypothesis of the generation and origin of auditory hallucinations is that they derive from inner speech that is misidentified as external speech because of defective self-monitoring.[10] Speech-relevant areas are predominantly located in the left hemisphere in right-handed individuals, which seems to be the more involved hemisphere in the generation of auditory hallucinations. The hypothesis for an association of speech-related circuits in the generation of auditory hallucinations is further supported by a decreased number of auditory hallucinations after application of repetitive transcranial magnetic stimulation over the left hemispheric temporoparietal cortex, disrupting neuronal activity between the stimulated brain area and remote regions.[11]

Prospects

In auditory hallucinations, pathological activated brain regions are mainly located in the frontal and temporal language and auditory areas. Common theories on schizophrenia propose a disruption in the frontotemporal networks.[12] These theories have received further support from recent electrophysiological studies. One functional study reported a lack of coherence in the brain electrical activity during speech in hallucinating patients, whereas coherence was observed in healthy controls.[13] The use of DTI allows the textural investigation of the underlying cerebral white matter microstructure. With DTI, it is possible to analyse the interconnection of the different brain regions that are involved in the generation of auditory hallucinations. The three most prominent fibre tracts that connect the anterior to the posterior part of the brain are the cingulate bundle, the arcuate fascicle (superior longitudinal fascicle), and the uncinate fascicle. A recent DTI study in schizophrenia showed a lack of left-greater-than-right asymmetry in the uncinate fascicle.[14] Furthermore, alterations in the long frontotemporal fibres, especially in the superior longitudinal fascicle, have been described to correlate significantly with normal human development.[15] Alteration in this location was found in children with dyslexia, indicating its importance for normal development of language functions.[16] The arcuate fascicle connects the frontal Broca's area with the temporoparietal Wernicke's area. In a recent study we could demonstrate alterations in the long fibre tracts connecting frontal with temporal brain regions, especially in the superior longitudinal fascicle, in schizophrenia patients with auditory hallucinations, indicating changes in connectivity between language related areas.[17]

Summary

The studies of the past decade uncovered relevant mechanisms responsible for the appearance of auditory hallucinations. Macroscopic structural studies found evidence of altered temporal lobe volume. Functional imaging studies broadened that knowledge and detected dysfunctions in the language and auditory areas, partly located in the altered temporal lobe. Research in the field of auditory hallucinations in schizophrenia on the basis of neuropsychological investigations and spatial and temporal high-resolution neurophysiological studies added the theory of a disruption of the frontotemporal connections which now could be demonstrated with MR-DTI.

References

1. Nayani TH, David AS, The auditory hallucination: a phenomenological survey. *Psychol Med* 1996; **26**:177–189.
2. Southard EE, On the topographic distribution of cortex lesions and anomalies in dementia praecox with some account of their functional significance. *Am J Insanity* 1915; **71**:671.
3. Shapleske J, Rossell SL, Simmons A, David AS, Woodruff PW, Are auditory hallucinations the consequence of abnormal cerebral lateralization? A morphometric

MRI study of the sylvian fissure and planum temporale. *Biol Psychiatry* 2001; **49**:685–693.

4. Ogawa S, Lee TM, Kay AR, Tank DW, Brain magnetic resonance imaging with contrast dependent on blood oxygenation. *Proc Natl Acad Sci USA* 1990; **87**:9868–9872.

5. Basser PJ, Mattiello J, LeBihan D, MR diffusion tensor spectroscopy and imaging. *Biophys J* 1994; **66**:259–267.

6. Weiss AP, Heckers S, Neuroimaging of hallucinations: a review of the literature. *Psychiatry Res* 1999; **92**:61–74.

7. Silbersweig DA, Stern E, Frith C et al, A functional neuroanatomy of hallucinations in schizophrenia. *Nature* 1995; **378**:176–179.

8. Dierks T, Linden DE, Jandl M et al, Activation of Heschl's gyrus during auditory hallucinations. *Neuron* 1999; **22**:615–621.

9. David AS, Woodruff PW, Howard R et al, Auditory hallucinations inhibit exogenous activation of auditory association cortex. *Neuroreport* 1996; **7**:932–936.

10. McGuire PK, Silbersweig DA, Wright I et al, Abnormal monitoring of inner speech: a physiological basis for auditory hallucinations. *Lancet* 1995; **346**:596–600.

11. Hoffman RE, Hawkins KA, Gueorguieva R et al, Transcranial magnetic stimulation of left temporoparietal cortex and medication-resistant auditory hallucinations. *Arch Gen Psychiatry* 2003; **60**:49–56.

12. Frith CD, Friston KJ, Herold S et al, Regional brain activity in chronic schizophrenic patients during the performance of a verbal fluency task. *Br J Psychiatry* 1995; **167**:343–349.

13. Ford JM, Mathalon DH, Whitfield S, Faustman WO, Roth WT, Reduced communication between frontal and temporal lobes during talking in schizophrenia. *Biol Psychiatry* 2002; **51**:485–492.

14. Kubicki M, Westin CF, Maier SE et al, Uncinate fasciculus findings in schizophrenia: a magnetic resonance diffusion tensor imaging study. *Am J Psychiatry* 2002; **159**:813–820.

15. Paus T, Zijdenbos A, Worsley K et al, Structural maturation of neural pathways in children and adolescents: in vivo study. *Science* 1999; **283**:1908–1911.

16. Klingberg T, Hedehus M, Temple E et al, Microstructure of temporo-parietal white matter as a basis for reading ability: evidence from diffusion tensor magnetic resonance imaging. *Neuron* 2000; **25**:493–500.

17. Hubl D, Koenig T, Strik W et al, Pathways that make voices: white matter changes in auditory hallucinations. *Arch Gen Psych* 2004 (in press).

chapter 3

Can we find the genes that predispose to schizophrenia?

Nadine Norton and Michael J Owen

The search for genes for schizophrenia has often been described as a 'search for the Holy Grail', implying, we assume, that it is a poetic and romantic quest for a single object of great significance but one that is ultimately doomed to failure. The purpose of this chapter is to show that, while the search may well be poetic and romantic, there is no single prize of great significance. Rather, there are several and possibly many prizes each of which will help unlock the secrets of schizophrenia. The quest for these, while difficult, is not doomed to failure and at last seems to be showing clear signs of success.

It is well known from genetic epidemiological studies that schizophrenia runs in families. Moreover, an impressive body of evidence from twin and adoption studies shows that individual differences in liability are largely genetic with heritability estimates close to 0.8. However, finding disease genes has proved difficult because both the phenotype and genotype are complex and poorly understood. Schizophrenia is a syndrome that may contain a number of different disorders each reflecting different pathogenic processes. We still understand little about its pathophysiology and cannot predict with any degree of certainty the likely function of the genes we expect to find. Finally, genetic epidemiology suggests that the mode of transmission is likely to be complex such that we are dealing with multiple genes rather than genes of large effect. Genes that increase the risk in siblings by greater than 3 are unlikely and most of the genes are going to be of relatively small effect, possibly with exceptions in some isolated or particularly high density families. The problem is that although we can say that genes are important and that there are likely to be a number of them involved, we cannot say how many there are, how much risk each one confers or how much they interact.

Faced with a complex syndrome of unknown genetic architecture, it is a useful exercise to consider what we might expect to find on the basis of genetic epidemiology and from findings in other complex traits especially in animals where genetic studies are more advanced. First, it is likely that there are a number of genes of modest effect (oligogenes), but that there will also almost certainly be a huge number of genes of small effect (polygenes) that are influencing susceptibility and modifying the phenotype. As a result we can expect a great deal of complexity and uncertainty in terms of the predictive value of genetics. Second, given the fact that schizophrenia is defined only at a syndromic level, heterogeneity is expected. It should also be no surprise if schizophrenia and bipolar disorder have some genes in common, given the clinical overlap of the two syndromes. Third, one might hope to be able to identify intermediate phenotypes, i.e. phenotypes that lie on the pathway between genes and the clinical phenotype in the way that plasma lipid levels and blood pressure lie between the genes and the clinical phenotype of ischaemic vascular disease. Fourth, gene–environment and gene–gene interactions should also be expected, and data from animal work suggest that these can be common and complex. One such example is bristle number in *Drosophila*, whereby the same allele that increases bristle number in males also decreases it in females, suggesting quite subtle and complex effects at the level of the genome.[1] Fifth, complex traits in animals are often associated, not with genetic variants altering the physical structure of the protein, but with those that alter the way in which the gene is expressed. These can be very hard to find, as they are often located outside the coding sequence of the gene and sometimes some distance from it. Finally, in many instances, allelic heterogeneity is present and it may well be that the schizophrenia risk depends not just on the inheritance of a single allele at a particular single polymorphic site, but as a read out of a whole number of polymorphic sites across a susceptibility gene.

The main methods used to search for susceptibility genes for schizophrenia have been linkage and association and the study of chromosomal abnormalities. Despite difficulties, progress has been made in each of these areas.

Linkage studies

Early linkage studies clearly excluded the hypothesis that single-gene forms of the disorder exist such as are seen in Alzheimer's disease and breast cancer. The results of linkage studies of schizophrenia have seemed to some to be disappointing with positive studies often falling short of being compelling and failures to replicate being abundant. However, as more than 20 genome-wide studies have been reported and as sample sizes and hence power have increased, so replicated, positive linkages to several chromosomal regions have accumulated (Figure 3.1). Three of the best-supported

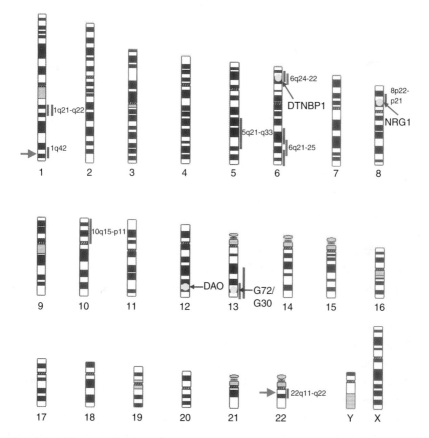

Figure 3.1 *Ideogram showing major chromosomal regions implicated by linkage studies of schizophrenia. Blue lines indicate areas for which suggestive evidence of linkage has been found in more than one data set. Red lines indicate regions where evidence of linkage has achieved genome-wide significance. Red arrows indicate site of chromosomal abnormalities associated with schizophrenia. Yellow circles indicate the location of genes implicated as possible schizophrenia susceptibility loci.*

regions are 6p24-22, 1q21-22 and 13q32-34. In these cases single studies achieved genome-wide significance at p < 0.05, that is, a linkage value that is expected less than once by chance in 20 complete genome scans. Moreover, in each case suggestive positive findings have also been reported in other samples. In two further regions several groups have reported highly suggestive evidence for linkage. These are 8p21-22 and 6q21-25. Other promising regions in which positive findings have been obtained from more than one study include 22q11-12, 5q21-q33, 10p15-p11 and 1q42.

Chromosomal abnormalities

There have been numerous reports of associations between schizophrenia and chromosomal abnormalities, but with two exceptions none has as yet provided convincing evidence to support the location of a gene conferring risk for schizophrenia. The first of these exceptions is the association with velocardiofacial syndrome (VCFS), a disorder caused by deletions of chromosome 22q11. This occurs in 1/4000 live births and results in a complex phenotype with multiple congenital abnormalities, characteristic dysmorphology, cleft palate, cardiac defects, learning disabilities and high rates of psychiatric disorder. Rate of schizophrenia in adults carrying the deletion is as high as 24%.[2] The fact that a number of linkage studies have also implicated 22q11 suggests that a gene within the deleted region might also be involved more generally in susceptibility to schizophrenia. The second is from a large Scottish family with 47% prevalence of mental illnesses including schizophrenia. A balanced reciprocal translocation between chromosomes 1 and 11 co-segregated with illness. Subsequent mapping of the translocation breakpoint has identified three disrupted genes on chromosome 1 and studies are now beginning to identify the pathways that are implicated by these genes.[3,4]

Association studies

Most association studies have looked at functional candidate genes such as neurotransmitter receptors and a limited number of neurodevelopmental genes. There have been many positive claims but no clear replicated findings. A number of reasons exist as to why one might expect to get both false positives and false negatives. However, it is of greater interest that a number of positive studies over the past 12 months have provided evidence for association with positional candidate genes, i.e. genes that are located within regions of genetic linkage. The Icelandic deCODE genetics group showed association of the *neuregulin 1* (*NRG1*) gene (located on chromosome 8p22-p21) to schizophrenia, identifying a significant core haplotype for disease susceptibility (relative risk 2.1)[5] and this finding has since been replicated in a Scottish population.[6] A second positive association has come from the *dysbindin* (*DTNBP1*) gene on chromosome 6p. Initial association was with a rare haplotype in Irish families[7] and replication has since been achieved in a German population.[8] The gene *G72* (chromosome 13q22-34) is also associated with schizophrenia and interaction analysis has shown that *G72* interacts with a second gene, DAO (D-amino acid oxidase), which itself is associated with the disorder. Further analysis has revealed that combinations of *G72/DAO* genotypes have a synergistic effect on disease risk.[9] These findings have in common the fact that all three genes were identified by detailed characterization of linked regions. They are also all of association with multiple non-coding variants in the form of haplotypes rather than with individual markers. Further work remains to be done before we understand precisely how genetic variation at each locus confers susceptibility and protection. Moreover, in each case the relative risk is small (< 2.5) and cannot fully explain the linkage finding in the relevant region. These observations could suggest that the associated polymorphisms/haplotypes are in linkage disequilibrium with pathogenic variants elsewhere in the associated gene or in a neighbouring gene. Alternatively, association may arise not from a single variation in the relevant gene but from the combined effect of several different variants. It is also possible that the respective linkages reflect variation at two or more linked loci.

Will genetics pay off?

Schizophrenia has substantial heritability and understanding its causes is likely to be difficult if not impossible without finding the genes implicated. Despite a number of obstacles there are now promising data to support several chromosomal regions and genes. These successes are immensely encouraging. The existence of several promising linked regions suggests that other susceptibility genes for schizophrenia are likely to be found in the coming years. The ability of genetics to implicate novel genes and pathways in the pathogenesis of schizophrenia has already opened up new vistas for neurobiological research[10] and we can expect more in the coming years. However, we must continue to expect complexities: complexity at the level of the genome, with many genes involved, at the level of the gene, with many polymorphisms within individual genes involved, and at the level of gene–environment interaction. In spite of this, with technical advances in genomics and current knowledge there are grounds for optimism.

References

1. Nuzhdin SV, Dilda CL, Mackay TF, The genetic architecture of selection response. Inferences from fine-scale mapping of bristle number quantitative trait loci in *Drosophila melanogaster. Genetics* 1999; **153**:1317–1331.
2. Murphy KC, Owen MJ, Velo-cardio-facial syndrome (VCFS): a model for understanding the genetics and pathogenesis of schizophrenia. *Br J Psychiatry* 2001; **179**:397–402.
3. Millar JK, Wilson-Annan JC, Anderson S et al, Disruption of two novel genes by a translocation co-segregating with schizophrenia. *Hum Mol Genet* 2000; **9**:1415–1423.
4. Ozeki Y, Tomoda T, Kleiderlein J et al, Disrupted-in-Schizophrenia-1 (DISC-1): mutant truncation prevents binding to NudE-like (NUDEL) and inhibits neurite outgrowth. *Proc Natl Acad Sci USA* 2003; **100**:289–294.
5. Stefansson H, Sigurdsson E, Steinthorsdottir V et al, Neuregulin 1 and susceptibility to schizophrenia. *Am J Hum Genet* 2002; **71**:877–892.
6. Stefansson H, Sarginson J, Kong A et al, Association of neuregulin 1 with schizophrenia confirmed in a Scottish population. *Am J Hum Genet* 2003; **72**:83–87.
7. Straub RE, Jiang Y, MacLean CJ et al, Genetic variation in the 6p22.3 gene DTNBP1, the human ortholog of the mouse dysbindin gene, is associated with schizophrenia. *Am J Hum Genet* 2002; **71**:337–348.
8. Schwab SG, Knapp M, Mondabon S et al, Support for association of schizophrenia with genetic variation in the 6p22.3 gene, dysbindin, in sib-pair families with linkage and in an additional sample of triad families. *Am J Hum Genet* 2003; **72**:185–190.
9. Chumakov I, Blumenfeld M, Guerassimenko O et al, Genetic and physiological data implicating the new human gene G72 and the gene for D-amino acid oxidase in schizophrenia. *Proc Natl Acad Sci USA* 2002; **99**:13675–13680.
10. Harrison PJ, Owen MJ, Genes for schizophrenia? Recent findings and their pathological implications. *Lancet* 2003; **361**:417–419.

chapter 4

Genes for schizophrenia can be detected – data from Iceland implicates *neuregulin 1*

Hannes Petursson, Hreinn Stefansson, Engilbert Sigurdsson, Valgerdur Steinthorsdottir, Thordur Sigmundsson, Jon Brynjolfsson, Steinunn Gunnarsdottir, Omar Ivarsson, Omar Hjaltason, Helgi Jonsson, Vala G Gudnadottir, Elsa Gudmundsdottir, Brynjolfur Ingvarsson, Andres Ingason, Sigmundur Sigfusson, Hronn Hardardottir, Jeffrey R Gulcher and Kari Stefansson

There have been a number of genome-wide linkage scans over the past several years with at least a modest evidence of linkage on 1q, 2 and 22q and more recently good evidence for location of genes on chromosomes 6, 12 and 13q. Linkage on chromosome 8p has also been suggested by a number of workers studying different populations.[1-8] We initially collected 110 patients from 33 families for which affected individuals within a family could be as distantly related as second cousins (further details on methodology are described in the Appendix on p. 28). In the genomewide scan 950 framework microsatellite markers were employed using genotyping conditions and protocols described elsewhere.[9] Of the 110 affected individuals in the 33 families, 106 were available for genotyping (102 schizophrenia patients, three diagnosed with unspecified functional psychosis and one with schizo-affective disorder). The analysis was based on a model-free, multi-point, allele-sharing approach. The scan revealed suggestive or supportive evidence for linkage on six chromosomes where the LOD score was higher than one, i.e. on chromosomes 1, 3, 6, 8, 14 and on chromosome X. The most prominent peak in this study was on chromosome 8p, which overlapped with a previously reported locus, although it appeared that our peak was 10 to 15 cM centromeric to the results of some of the other studies. This may be explained by differences in the density and order of markers or our locus may be a distinct locus.

The 8p locus was fine-mapped with additional markers at a marker distance of about 100–150 kb (kilobases) over a 30 cM region. We used a subset of the markers for linkage analysis, avoiding markers in linkage disequilibrium, which then increased the information content from 0.7 to 0.9. The LOD score declined from 3.06 to 2.53 and the results were, thus, only suggestive of linkage to 8p, but along with results of previous studies they were considered sufficiently convincing to start a search for haplotypes. Further markers were

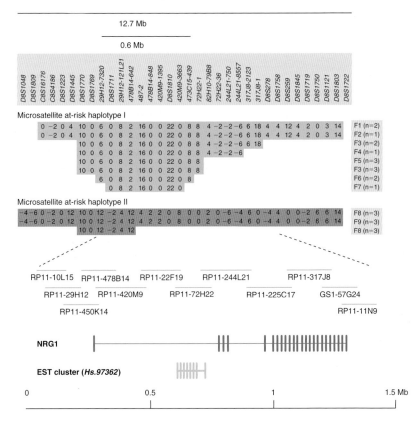

Figure 4.1 Microsatellite at-risk haplotypes on chromosome 8p and known genes within a region showing haplotype sharing (Reproduced from Stefansson et al. Am J Hum Genet 2002; *71*:877–892)[10] (with permission of the University of Chicago Press). © 2002 by The American Society of Human Genetics. All rights reserved.

added which were spaced at about 75 kb over a 5 cM region. Haplotypes shared between families, haplotype I and haplotype II (Figure 4.1), caught our attention as the shared haplotypes span up to 13 Mb. There were 15 individuals from seven of the 33 linkage families that shared at-risk haplotype I, and nine individuals from two families on the haplotype II, which is substantially rarer than the first. Exact marker locations and order were established with bacterial artificial chromosome clones (BACs). At this stage 373 more patients were included for association analysis. The refined haplotype analysis revealed that the at-risk haplotype sat right on top of two genes, the *neuregulin 1* gene and a cluster of expressed sequence tags (EST) with unknown function. The work then proceeded to sequence the mouse locus in order to help identify exons and promoter regions. Twenty-five exons were found in the *neuregulin 1* gene, some of these were novel and eight exons were found for the EST cluster.

Moving to single nucleotide polymorphism (SNP) analysis, all coding SNPs were genotyped and a number of SNPs in promoter regions and also some in conserved regions were genotyped. All patients were genotyped for 58 SNPs and a subgroup of 94 patients and 124 controls were also genotyped for an additional 123 SNPs, altogether 181 SNPs were genotyped. This then revealed that haplotype I had the same SNP core haplotype as other microsatellite haplotypes which were in slight excess in patients (Figure 4.2). Initially it was considered that these haplotypes were separate, independent

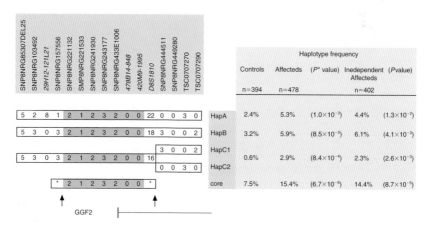

Figure 4.2 *Microsatellite and SNP at-risk haplotypes at the 5′ end of the* NRG1 *gene (Reproduced from Stefansson et al. Am J Hum Genet 2002; **71**:877–892)[10] (with permission of the University of Chicago Press). © 2002 by The American Society of Human Genetics. All rights reserved.*

haplotypes, and it was not until somewhat later that it became evident that they all share a 7-allele core at-risk haplotype. The core haplotype spans 290 kb. Linkage disequilibrium is prominent in this area and therefore a haplotype based on a subset of the markers can be used as a surrogate to identify the 7-marker core at-risk haplotype.[10]

None of the core SNPs accounts for the same degree of association as well as the 7-allele haplotype and the SNP alleles are therefore not likely to be the causative variant. Transmission disequilibrium tests (TDTs) were performed in 50 schizophrenia trios where parents were heterozygous for the at-risk haplotype and in 33 instances the haplotype was transmitted and in 17 it was not. The difference is about two-fold, which is somewhat encouraging in view of the fact that the relative risk ratio for the core haplotype is 2.1. The core at-risk haplotype is found in 7.5% of normal controls and in 15.4% of all patients. Excluding the ones that are known to be related within four meiotic events, the frequency is 14.4%.

The next question is whether this association is found outside Iceland. There are collaborative replication studies ongoing, one with David St Clair at the University of Aberdeen, who has been studying schizophrenia for a number of years, the work being sponsored by Glaxo SmithKline. The findings in Iceland and Scotland are very similar. The frequency of the 7-marker haplotype in Scotland is 5.9% in controls, 10.2% in patients and the relative risk ratio is 1.8. In Iceland the frequencies are 7.6% and 14.4%, respectively and the relative risk ratio is 2.1. A significant difference is also demonstrated between affecteds and controls in both Scotland and Iceland when analysing the 5-marker SNP haplotype alone.

It is also encouraging that other genes are being identified, and may even act partly through common pathways. Regulation of glutamate signalling through the *N*-methyl-D-aspartate (NMDA) receptor pathway by *G72* interacting with the gene for D-amino acid oxidase (DAAO) has been reported by Chumakov and associates.[11] Dysbindin may also affect susceptibility to schizophrenia via the NMDA receptors.[12] *Neuregulin 1* also interacts with NMDA receptors affecting activation of neurotransmitters and glutamate transmission.

Functional studies have found that mutant mice heterozygous for either *neuregulin 1* or *ErbB4* show a behavioural phenotype that overlaps with mouse models of schizophrenia. Furthermore, *neuregulin 1* hypomorphs have fewer functional NMDA receptors than wild type mice. The behavioural phenotypes of the *neuregulin 1* hypomorphs are partially reversible with clozapine.[10]

It is possible that these findings are indicative of glutamate dysfunction, taking into consideration that glutamate signalling through the NMDA receptor may induce psychosis in healthy people and exacerbate manifestations of schizophrenia. Decreased binding to and expression of subunits of glutamate receptors occur in schizophrenia patients. Clozapine facilitates glutamate transmission by increasing NMDA receptor expression. Reduced numbers of NMDA receptors result in behavioural discrepancies similar to those produced by NMDA antagonists which may be reversible with clozapine. However, in view of the numerous reciprocal synaptic relationships it becomes obvious that the dopamine and glutamate dysfunction hypotheses are not incompatible.

Conclusion

Neuregulin 1 was identified as a susceptibility gene for schizophrenia by standard operational protocols for positional cloning. Association has been confirmed in a large case–control replication study in more than 600 Scottish patients and controls genotyped for the at-risk haplotype markers. Behavioural and pharmacological data on mouse mutants of *neuregulin 1* and *ErbB4*, as well as glutamate receptor binding data, support the role of *neuregulin 1* in schizophrenia. However, in spite of finding more than 1200 SNPs in the *neuregulin 1* gene and scoring 181 of them for association, we have not yet found a clear pathogenic mutation, which may in fact be the case for common disorders in general. If *neuregulin 1* is a schizophrenia susceptibility gene, its impact is unlikely to be limited to Icelandic or Scottish populations since schizophrenia has also been linked to chromosome 8 in other populations. Further collaborative studies are under way to explore this.

Finally, although the findings presented in this chapter are promising, it is prudent to urge caution and further research to establish unequivocal replications. Attempts at replication may be confounded by the finding of different alleles or haplotypes. It is imperative to continue the search for other schizophrenia susceptibility genes. The study of potential endophenotypes as well as the overlap between schizophrenia and bipolar disorders may provide further clues to the pathophysiology of schizophrenia and related disorders.

Appendix

The work presented in this chapter has been ongoing for the past 5 years in collaboration with deCODE genetics in Reykjavik, Hoffman La Roche in Basel and colleagues at all three psychiatric departments in Iceland. Functional and replication studies are being conducted in collaboration with research groups in different countries.[10,13] The research was approved by appropriate ethics committees. The Data Protection Commission (DPC) in Iceland has overseen this work like all other projects that deCODE undertakes in Iceland. All personal identifiers were encrypted by the DPC with a third party encryption system.[14] Researchers at deCODE did not have access to personally identifiable data and similarly clinicians were unaware of individual genotypic data. An extensive genealogy database which is encrypted in the same manner was used for clustering patients in families for linkage analysis. The database contains genealogy information back to the settlement of Iceland. It is particularly valuable for psychiatric diseases since phenotype information in psychiatry can go far back, information from church registries could even be used, as persons needing community support were registered for centuries. Thus, founder pedigrees can be analysed using information from church registers for people deceased long ago. In this study the probands were identified via referrals to inpatient and outpatient services of the psychiatric departments in Iceland. For this particular part of the work 476 patients were recruited, comprising 440 with schizophrenia, 32 with schizo-affective disorder and four with unspecified functional psychosis. The diagnoses were made according to the Research Diagnostic Criteria (RDC)[15] and the lifetime version of the Schizophrenia and Affective Disorder Schedule (SADS-L) was used.[16] Psychiatrists were blind to genotypic data and made consensus diagnoses.

References

1. Pulver AE, Lasseter VK, Kasch L et al, Schizophrenia: a genome scan targets chromosomes 3p and 8p as potential sites of susceptibility genes. *Am J Med Genet* 1995; **60**:252–260.
2. Kendler KS, MacLean CJ, O'Neill FA et al, Evidence for a schizophrenia vulnerability locus on chromosome 8p in the Irish study of high-density schizophrenia families. *Am J Psychiatry* 1996; **153**:1534–1540.
3. Levinson DF, Wildenauer DB, Schwab SG et al, Additional support for schizophrenia linkage on chromosomes 6 and 8: a multicenter study. *Am J Med Genet* 1996; **67**:580–594.
4. Blouin JL, Dombroski BA, Nath SK et al, Schizophrenia susceptibility loci on chromosomes 13q32 and 8p21. *Nat Genet* 1998; **20**:70–73.

5. Kaufmann CA, Suarez B, Malaspina D et al, NIMH genetics initiative millennium schizophrenia consortium: linkage analysis of African-American pedigrees. *Am J Med Genet* 1998; **81**:282–289.

6. Shaw SH, Kelly M, Smith AB et al, A genome-wide search for schizophrenia susceptibility genes. *Am J Med Genet* 1998; **81**:364–376.

7. Brzustowicz LM, Honer WG, Chow EW et al, Linkage of familial schizophrenia to chromosome 13q32. *Am J Hum Genet* 1999; **65**:1096–1103.

8. Gurling HM, Kalsi G, Brynjolfsson J et al, Genomewide genetic linkage analysis confirms the presence of susceptibility loci for schizophrenia, on chromosomes 1q32.2, 5q33.2 and 8p21-22 and provides support for linkage to schizophrenia, on chromosomes 11q23.3-24 and 20q12.1-11.23. *Am J Hum Genet* 2001; **68**:661–673.

9. Gretarsdottir S, Sveinbjornsdottir S, Jonsson HH et al, Localization of a susceptibility gene for common forms of stroke to 5q12. *Am J Hum Genet* 2002; **70**:593–603.

10. Stefansson H, Sigurdsson E, Steinthorsdottir V et al, *Neuregulin 1* and susceptibility to schizophrenia. *Am J Hum Genet* 2002; **71**:877–892.

11. Chumakov I, Blumenfeld M, Guerassimenko O et al, Genetic and physiological data implicating the new human gene *G72* and the gene for D-amino acid oxidase in schizophrenia. *Proc Natl Acad Sci USA* 2002; **99**:13675–13680.

12. Straub RE, MacLean CJ, Ma Y et al, Genome-wide scans of three independent sets of 90 Irish multiplex schizophrenia families and follow-up of selected regions in all families provides evidence for multiple susceptibility genes. *Mol Psychiatry* 2002; **7**:542–559.

13. Stefansson H, Sarginson J, Kong A et al, Association of *neuregulin 1* with schizophrenia confirmed in a Scottish population. *Am J Hum Genet* 2003; **72**: 83–87.

14. Gulcher JR, Kristjansson K, Gudbjartsson H et al, Protection of privacy by third-party encryption in genetic research in Iceland. *Eur J Hum Genet* 2000; **8**:739–742.

15. Spitzer RL, Endicott J, Robins E, Research diagnostic criteria: rationale and reliability. *Arch Gen Psychiatry* 1978; **35**:773–782.

16. Spitzer R, Endicott J (eds), *The schedule for affective disorders and schizophrenia, lifetime version.* 3rd edn. New York State Psychiatric Institute: New York, 1977.

chapter 5

Pharmacogenetics is the real future of genetic research in schizophrenia

Dalu Mancama, Maria J Arranz and Robert W Kerwin

Advances in drug design and development have brought about substantial improvements in the clinical management of patients. However, not all individuals benefit from pharmacological intervention as some fail to respond satisfactorily while others develop side effects that impair the overall success of treatment. This variable outcome is widely recognized as a significant problem throughout clinical practice. Its reasons began to be better understood in the 1950s, when the relation between inherited differences among individuals and therapeutic outcome was identified. During this period researchers first described the association between prolonged muscle relaxation after suxamethonium administration and an inherited deficiency in plasma cholinesterase,[1] and linked haemolysis during antimalarial treatment to inherited levels of the enzyme glucose 6-phosphate dehydrogenase.[2] The clinical implications of these discoveries heralded the inception of pharmacogenetics, and led to early studies examining the influence of genetic polymorphisms on enzyme activity, and determining how these relate to the therapeutic effects of clinical compounds.

Pharmacogenetics has now become a major scientific discipline, and has established itself at the forefront of research in schizophrenia. The aetiology of schizophrenia remains unclear but a participation of aberrant neurotransmitter signalling has been proposed, and this contribution has been substantiated by the development of antipsychotic drugs that selectively target neurotransmitter receptor sites and effectively alleviate many of the disorder's symptoms. However, up to 50% of patients remain refractory to treatment, while others react adversely,[3] and this frequently necessitates switching between drug regimes in a patient in an attempt to find the most suitable option. This often leads to episodes of exacerbated symptomatology while a more suitable drug is sought, whereas delays in identifying the most effective alternative often have long-term consequences on future outcome. Several variables, including gender, age of onset of illness, symptom type, and drug-related adverse effects such as extrapyramidal symptoms and weight gain, have been proposed as indicators of antipsychotic outcome.[4,5] However, many of these remain to be validated, and furthermore, are of limited clinical value as most are only useful once treatment has already begun. At present therefore no validated approach exists for accurately selecting the most effective antipsychotic a priori.

Today potential inherited differences in drug-metabolizing enzymes, drug transporters, and receptors to influence drug efficacy are well recognized. Despite this, the extent to which inherited differences influence antipsychotic outcome remains to be determined. Thus, although concordance for outcome to these drugs has been demonstrated among twins in case studies,[6-8] further larger studies are required to establish the precise magnitude of this contribution. Notwithstanding this a strong genetic component is proposed, and pharmacogenetics has been instrumental in attempting to identify the participating genes. Not surprisingly the potential influence of neurotransmitter receptors has formed the focus of much of this work, since these sites are implicated in the aetiology of psychosis and represent the primary targets of antipsychotic action. Genetic alterations, including those that potentially alter receptor binding, expression and distribution, have been identified throughout these candidates and examined through association studies to identify important variants. This has led to the identification of dopaminergic and serotonergic pathway variants that may be important to drug response, and to antipsychotic-related adverse responses such as tardive dyskinesia and weight gain. Similar variants influencing drug metabolism and other aspects of antipsychotic action have, until recently, remained largely uninvestigated, but the potential benefits of such work are well recognized and comprehensive findings are soon expected from this area. The advent of whole genome mapping has brought with it significant advances for pharmacogenetics. The field now bears far reaching implications for schizophrenia research, where the identification of genes important to antipsychotic action is expected to facilitate the development of future drug prescribing strategies. Ultimately, pharmacogenetics will enable substantial improvements in the design and development of these drugs, while reducing the adverse effects associated with their use. This chapter examines the impact of pharmacogenetics on schizophrenia research, and explores its future role in our understanding and treatment of the disorder.

What influences antipsychotic outcome?

The combined use of drug and social therapies is considered the most effective strategy for treating schizophrenia. However, it is the use of antipsychotics that has proved particularly beneficial for alleviating many of the symptoms of the disorder. Despite their proven potency, a high proportion of patients fail to respond to antipsychotic treatment while a similar number develop potentially serious side effects.[3] A compelling need has therefore arisen to identify the reasons underlying this heterogeneous outcome. The potential of environmental factors such as co-medication, patient lifestyle, and compliance, to influence treatment has long been known and is widely acknowledged. However, these factors do not considerably account for the variability in outcome seen with antipsychotics. In recent years the link between inherited differences and treatment outcome has become unequivocal, and this relation is now considered the most likely explanation for the variability seen in antipsychotic outcome. In particular, inherited differences in drug metabolism, drug transportation and site of action of drug have been implicated, and these mechanisms have subsequently become the major focus of pharmacogenetic studies in schizophrenia.

Antipsychotic drug metabolism

The primary role of drug metabolism is to facilitate the deactivation and excretion of pharmacologically active compounds from the body. This is mediated by specific enzymes that catalyse either phase I or phase II reactions. Phase I enzymes catalyse drug biotransformation by oxidation, reduction or hydrolysis, while phase II enzymes couple a drug to an endogenous compound (such as glycine or glutathionine) to render it inactive.[9] Antipsychotic compounds undergo extensive drug metabolism, and in the majority of cases this is mediated by one or a combination of the cytochrome P450 (CYP) enzymes.[10] More than 30 different isoforms are known, though only CYP1A2, CYP2C19, CYP2D6 and CYP3A4 are considered relevant to antipsychotic metabolism. Clozapine, for example, is metabolized by CYP1A2, together with a minor contribution from CYP3A4,

CYP2C19, and CYP2D6, while for quetiapine and ziprasidone the principal enzyme is CYP3A4.[11] The phenotypic consequences of *CYP* polymorphisms were first highlighted for CYP2D6 in which a recessive functional variant, prevalent in approximately 7% of Caucasian populations, was linked to deficient debrisoquine metabolism.[12] Subsequently more than 70 such variants have been identified of which at least 15 encode non-functional gene products. Depending on the variant type and number inherited, individuals are poor metabolizers, extensive metabolizers or ultrarapid metabolizers of substrates of CYP2D6. Similar phenotypic differences have been described for CYP2C19, while the full extent to which polymorphisms in CYP1A2, CYP2A6 and CYP3A4 influence activity remains to be clarified. The consequences of altered enzyme activity are varied, but can often lead to acute drug toxicity, or can influence treatment efficacy by modifying the relationship between drug dose and plasma concentration. These ramifications have led to the development of pharmacogenetic strategies on antipsychotic action to identify heritable differences in enzyme activity that are relevant to this form of treatment.

Pharmacogenetics of antipsychotic metabolism

The potential for enzyme alterations to influence antipsychotic metabolism has formed the focus of a number of recent studies, through which relationships have been identified between alterations in CYP1A2 and CYP2D6 activity, for example, and steady-state plasma levels of clozapine and its metabolite norclozapine, and risperidone, respectively.[13–15] However the influence these bear in relation to drug efficacy remains to be comprehensively examined, though some case studies have reported a contribution of CYP1A2 variants in determining the final outcome of clozapine response.[16,17] Clozapine is partly metabolized by CYP2D6, but functionally important variants of this enzyme do not appear to be influential,[18] while the participation of CYP2C19 and CYP3A4 remains to be determined for these drugs.

In contrast to phase I reaction enzymes, less is known regarding the extent to which phase II enzymes such as *N*-acetyltransferases and methyltransferases participate in antipsychotic metabolism. While this remains to be determined, polymorphisms that alter activity have already been identified for some of these proteins,[19,20] and the examination of those variants pertinent to antipsychotic action represents a potential area of focus for future studies. The contribution of such variants to treatment-related side effects is another area where future investigation is expected to prove beneficial.

Already significant associations have been reported between variants of CYP2D6 and CYP1A2, and susceptibility to antipsychotic-induced movement disorders such as tardive dyskinesia,[21,22] but extensive work is still required to validate these findings and exploit their clinical relevance.

Mechanisms of antipsychotic drug action

Although inherited pharmacokinetic traits may be important in determining antipsychotic outcome, similar changes at the site of drug action are thought to play a large role in determining the final efficacy to these drugs. The efficacy of the first widely available antipsychotic, chlorpromazine, was found to involve dopamine receptor DRD_2 blockade, and this knowledge facilitated the development of other compounds such as haloperidol that possess high DRD_2 antagonism.[10] Despite this property these compounds do not sufficiently alleviate the spectrum of symptoms that characterize schizophrenia, and up to 50% of patients remain refractory to treatment while others develop severe extrapyramidal side effects. This shortcoming has spurred the development of atypical antipsychotics, which elicit their efficacy through dopamine receptor DRD_2 and serotonin $5\text{-}HT_{2A}$ receptor blockade while demonstrating a low propensity towards extrapyramidal symptoms.[23] The drugs also target other sites including the histamine 1 receptor, the muscarinic acetylcholine 1 receptor, serotonin $5\text{-}HT_{2C}$ and $5\text{-}HT_7$ receptors, dopamine receptors DRD_3 and DRD_4, and α-adrenergic α_1 receptors, as summarized in Table 5.1. The distinct receptor binding profile displayed by these drugs ultimately determines their unique therapeutic action, and to an extent the profile of side effects associated with their use. In recent years the availability of sequence data has enabled the screening for and subsequent identification of numerous gene variants, of which a proportion have been found that may influence the functional integrity of neurotransmitter pathways. These variants could be important in determining the efficacy of antipsychotic drugs, and this prospect has formed the focus of a number of recent studies.

Pharmacogenetics of antipsychotic action

Dopaminergic system

All antipsychotics exhibit moderate to high affinity for dopamine receptor binding sites, particularly DRD_2 and DRD_4, and much interest has been

Table 5.1 Human receptor binding affinities (Ki, nM) for antipsychotic drugs

	Haloperidol	Clozapine	Olanzapine	Risperidone	Quetiapine	Ziprasidone
D_1	120	29	52	580	1300	130
D_2	1.4	130	20	2.2	180	3.1
D_3	2.5	240	50	9.6	940	7.2
D_4	3.3	47	50	8.5	2200	32
5-HT_{1A}	3600	140	2100	210	230	2.5
$5\text{-HT}_{1D}{}^a$	>5000	1700	530	170	>5100	2.0
5-HT_{2A}	120	8.9	3.3	0.29	220	0.39
5-HT_{2C}	4700	17	10	10	1400	0.72
5-HT_6	6000	11	10	2000	4100	76
5-HT_7	1100	66	250	3.0	1800	9.6
H_1	44	1.8	2.8	19	8.7	47
$CHRM_1$	1600	1.8	4.7	2800	100	5100
α_1	4.7	4.0	54	1.4	15	13
α_2	1200	33	170	5.1	1000	310

aRepresent bovine affinities.
Binding affinities adapted from Schmidt AW et al. *Eur J Pharmacol* 2001; **425**:197–201.[24]

placed on determining the influence dopaminergic variants confer on drug outcome. Several important polymorphisms have been identified throughout these receptors, some of which alter receptor expression or binding and conceivably may influence treatment.[25] Studies of DRD$_4$ largely suggest that variants of this receptor do not, however, influence treatment response, at least in the case of clozapine treatment.[26–28] Studies to date have generally also not identified association between DRD$_2$ variants and response, though a DRD$_2$ *Taq I* polymorphism has been associated with short-term response to haloperidol.[29] A number of these polymorphisms have also been implicated in the aetiology of schizophrenia.[30,31] In contrast more interesting evidence has been reported for association between a DRD$_3$ Ser9Gly polymorphism and clozapine outcome, for which increased homozygosity for the Ser9 allele has been identified among poor responders.[32] This has been independently corroborated in other clozapine patients,[33] with a similar trend being reported elsewhere.[34] The relationship between Ser9Gly variants and response is further supported by a meta-analysis of these studies.[33] More recently strategies have been employed to investigate the influence of polymorphisms on specific symptoms of schizophrenia, and this has led to the identification of DRD_3 variants which influence improvements in positive symptoms following olanzapine treatment.[35] These findings, although tentative, support the role of dopaminergic blockade in antipsychotic action, and also give support to findings which implicate the role of such variants in the aetiology of schizophrenia.[36,37] Strong evidence of association has also been demonstrated between DRD_3 Ser9Gly variants and susceptibility to antipsychotic-induced tardive dyskinesia,[38-40] highlighting the potential influence of such variants in adverse drug responses.

Serotonergic system

Atypical antipsychotics possess high affinity for serotonergic receptors, particularly $5\text{-}HT_{2A}$, $5\text{-}HT_{2C}$ and $5\text{-}HT_6$, and conceivably inherited alterations in these may also be important for determining drug outcome. This contribution was confirmed when a $5\text{-}HT_{2A}$ 102-T/C polymorphism was found to be associated with clozapine response,[41] with comparable trends for association being independently observed in similar patient groups.[42-44] Meta-analysis of these and further studies subsequently confirmed this association.[45] Recently the 102-T/C polymorphism has also been associated with risperidone response.[46] Since the polymorphism is non-functional, studies have sought to identify other $5\text{-}HT_{2A}$ variants that are functional and associated with response. Such variants remain to be identified, although association with clozapine response has been reported for a $5\text{-}HT_{2A}$ (-1438-A/G) promoter polymorphism whose functional basis remains to be fully established.[45] A structural $5\text{-}HT_{2A}$ (His452Tyr) polymorphism has also been extensively studied for which the 452Tyr variant is associated with poor clozapine response.[43,45,47] Similar findings of association for clozapine have also been reported with a structural $5\text{-}HT_{2C}$ (Cys23Ser) polymorphism,[48] though other studies have as yet been unable to confirm this.[49] Work is also required to corroborate the association reported between a $5\text{-}HT_6$ (267-C/T) polymorphism and clozapine response.[50] Further to the contribution of serotonergic variants to drug response, studies have also sought to determine whether they may influence treatment-related side effects. Antipsychotic-induced weight gain has formed a particular focus of these studies, and the rationale for selecting these pathways arises from their pivotal role in regulating food intake and weight gain.[51] Initial studies did not identify any variants within $5\text{-}HT_{1A}$, $5\text{-}HT_{2A}$, and $5\text{-}HT_6$ that may be important,[52,53] although a trend for association was observed for the $5\text{-}HT_{2C}$ receptor.[52] More recent studies of this latter receptor have identified significant association between a $5\text{-}HT_{2C}$ (-759 C/T) polymorphism and clozapine-induced weight gain,[54,55] and work is ongoing to confirm this association and to identify further variants that are involved.

Influence of other systems

Pharmacogenetic studies in schizophrenia have traditionally focused on determining the contribution of dopaminergic and serotonergic variants in antipsychotic response and related side effects. However, these systems do not fully account for the variability observed in outcome to these drugs, and further candidates have been sought that might also be involved. These primarily constitute pathways mediating antipsychotic action, and include the α-adrenergic, histaminergic and muscarinic acetylcholine neurotransmitter systems. Antipsychotic drugs selectively target α_{1A} and α_{2A} receptors, although as yet few studies have examined their genetic contribution to treatment outcome. Several polymorphisms have been reported for these receptors,[56–58] and so far none of these has been found to be involved.[59] However, more comprehensive work in this area is required before the contribution of this system can be established. This is also the case for the histaminergic system. Clozapine, olanzapine and other antipsychotic drugs possess high affinity for the histamine 1 (H_1) receptor, and similar hypotheses have been put forward for the influence variants of this receptor may confer on treatment outcome. However, of the H_1 receptor polymorphisms that have been identified, none is associated with response. Similar variants within the histamine 2 (H_2) receptor have also been investigated, with evidence from two independent studies supporting a minor contribution to clozapine response of an H_2 receptor -1018-G/A promoter polymorphism.[60,61] Further work is required to clarify the nature of this relationship, and to determine the functional nature, if any, of this polymorphism. The muscarinic 1 receptor ($CHRM_1$) has also become a recent focus of studies, given the high affinity possessed for this target by antipsychotics. No relationship between $CHRM_1$ variants and therapeutic outcome has yet been found, although given the few studies that have been done further exploration in this area is necessary. Similar strategies of investigation remain to be extensively adopted for adverse responses to treatment that might be mediated by these aforementioned systems. These include hypotension and dizziness related to α-adrenergic blockade, weight gain and sedation related to histaminergic blockade, and hyposalivation and sinus tachycardia related to muscarinic blockade.[62]

Future role of pharmacogenetics in schizophrenia

Despite notable successes, the task of identifying the genes that influence antipsychotic outcome has so far proved arduous and has been met with somewhat limited success. Strategies for gene identification have largely been based on the candidate gene approach, which relies on prior knowledge of the aetiology of schizophrenia, and knowledge of the inherent pharmacological properties of antipsychotic drugs. However, the complex nature of antipsychotic action has proved a major challenge to this approach, primarily because at least several genes are thought to be involved and their identification has entailed screening large numbers of candidate genes at great effort, time and expense. Fortuitously, the advent of whole genome mapping has brought with it considerable advances in biomolecular technology, in particular, the development of microarray gene expression profiling. This large-scale pharmacogenomic strategy enables the screening of tens of thousands of genes in a relatively short period of time, and has already proved decisive in delineating novel biological processes related to asthma, cancer and inflammatory diseases such as rheumatoid arthritis.[63–65] Its application is expected to prove equally valuable in drug discovery and design.[66] Previously considered prohibitively expensive and unreliable, the availability of affordable kits combined with significant technical improvements has led to the widespread use of microarrays. They are now being incorporated into schizophrenia research and preliminary data have already been presented that may be pertinent to the disorder's underlying aetiology. These findings include the identification of genes involved in synaptic plasticity, neuronal development and postsynaptic signal transduction that may be important.[67–69] Similar scope exists for exploiting microarrays to provide a unique insight into the genes and pathways that influence antipsychotic outcome,[70,71] where the foremost goal will be to examine the effects of these compounds on neural activity and function. This strategy can further be applied to investigate simulation models of schizophrenia that employ psychomimetic drugs as a way of delineating the disorder's aetiology, as has recently been demonstrated with amphetamine and phencyclidine.[72,73] Novel candidate genes identified through this approach include transcription factors, metabolic enzymes and signal transduction genes. In addition, other genes have also been identified that bear no immediately apparent relation to schizophrenia or its treatment, and the significance of these remains to be determined. Advances in mutation detection technique now enable the rapid screening of all these candidate genes for polymorphisms of potential importance. This task is facilitated by the availability of large, publicly accessible databases that currently catalogue more than 3 million single nucleotide polymorphisms throughout the human genome.[74,75] Combined with the advances in genotyping technology that make analysis of these polymorphisms faster and cheaper, the application of these new technologies is expected to revolutionize the future identification of genes that contribute to the aetiology and treatment of schizophrenia.

A factor that has further complicated the identification of the participating genes stems from population differences in pharmacogenetic traits. This influence is exemplified by findings for treatment response to selective serotonin reuptake inhibitors (SSRIs), a class of antidepressants that mediate their actions by blocking serotonin transporter (5-HTT) action. The gene encoding the serotonin transporter contains a polymorphism of two common alleles (long and short) which differentially affect gene expression. Clear differences exist in the distribution of these alleles among populations. The long allele is associated with good response to SSRIs in Europeans,[76,77] while in Koreans and Japanese the opposite association has been observed.[78,79] Given the functional importance of these alleles, they would be expected to confer the same influence across these populations if they were the causative variant. Since this is not the case, it is possible that further pharmacologically important polymorphisms are yet to be discovered in this gene that confer opposite effects in Asian and European populations. While this remains to be established, these findings highlight the considerations posed by ethnic diversity on pharmacogenetic traits with a complex underlying basis.

A strategy that has been extensively adopted to facilitate gene identification is the incorporation of comprehensive clinical data in genetic studies that detail a wider spectrum of patient symptomatology, response outcome and treatment-related side effects. This contrasts with the approach of earlier studies that focused solely on the influence genes bear on general response. The incorporation of detailed clinical data has already proved effective in identifying genes involved in short-term response to haloperidol treatment and improvements in positive symptomatology during olanzapine treatment.[35,80] It has also facilitated the identification of genes that contribute to treatment-induced agranulocytosis, weight gain, tardive dyskinesia and neuroleptic malignant syndrome.[29,39,54] These findings currently remain to be comprehensively validated through large, prospective, independent studies. Furthermore, in their present form they lack clinical applicability, since individually they cannot accurately predict treatment outcome. A major goal of pharmacogenetics is to use this information to predict treatment outcome. The feasibility of this approach has already been demonstrated for the antipsychotic clozapine, for which a pertinent combination of gene variants have been used to successfully predict treatment response in approximately 76% of cases.[81] As further variants of importance are identified and incorporated into the predictive model, the accuracy of this test will improve to a clinically applicable level. Similar strategies are being developed for other widely prescribed antipsychotics including olanzapine and risperidone. Ultimately this work will lead to the development of gene-based diagnostic kits that are amenable for routine clinical use, and that tailor antipsychotic prescribing to the needs of each individual patient.

Conclusions

A major cause for concern in schizophrenia is the failure of patients to respond satisfactorily to antipsychotic medication while others experience adverse reactions associated with the use of these drugs. This heterogeneous outcome often impacts upon the long-term outlook of these individuals, while significantly increasing the social and financial costs associated with their care. A compelling need has arisen to identify the reasons underlying this variability, and in recent years pharmacogenetics has been at the forefront of research in schizophrenia to achieve this goal. This has facilitated the identification of genetic variants within dopaminergic and serotonergic pathways that contribute to antipsychotic response, and susceptibility to drugs-related side effects. Although the complex nature of antipsychotic action has impeded the identification of further genes of importance, advances in biomolecular technology now make this task more feasible. Comprehensive findings from such work are yet to be presented, but they are likely to prove decisive in the discovery of new drug targets, and in delineating the genetic aetiology of schizophrenia. This knowledge will be used to develop pharmacogenetic strategies that enable selection of the most effective drug on the basis of each patient's genetic profile, ultimately ensuring a dramatically improved level of treatment.

References

1. Kalow W, Familial incidence of low pseudocholinesterase level. *Lancet* 1956; **2**:576–577.
2. Carson PE, Flangan CL, Ickes CE, Alving AS, Enzymatic deficiency in primaquine sensitive erthrocytes. *Science* 1956; **124**:484–485.
3. Conley RR, Buchanan RW, Evaluation of treatment-resistant schizophrenia. *Schizophr Bull* 1997; **23**:663–674.
4. Lieberman JA, Koreen AR, Chakos M et al, Factors influencing treatment response and outcome of first-episode schizophrenia: implications for understanding the pathophysiology of schizophrenia. [Review] [43 refs]. *J Clin Psychiatry* 1996; **57**:Suppl 9.
5. Meltzer HY, Perry E, Jayathilake K, Clozapine-induced weight gain predicts improvement in psychopathology. *Schizophr Res* 2003; **59**:19–27.
6. Horácek J, Libiger J, Höschl C, Borzová K, Hendrychová I, Clozapine-induced concordant agranulocytosis in monozygotic twins. *Int J Psychiatry Clin Pract* 2001; **5**:71–73.
7. Mata I, Madoz V, Arranz MJ, Sham P, Murray RM, Olanzapine: concordant response in monozygotic twins with schizophrenia. *Br J Psychiatry* 2001; **178**:86.
8. Vojvoda D, Grimmell K, Sernyak M, Mazure CM, Monozygotic twins concordant for response to clozapine. *Lancet* 1996; **347**:61.
9. Weber WW, *Pharmacogenetics*. Oxford University Press: Oxford, 1997.
10. Ellenbroek BA, Cools AR, *Atypical Antipsychotics. Milestones in Drug Therapy*. Verlag AG, Publ: Birkhäuser, 2000.
11. Prior TI, Baker GB, Interactions between the cytochrome P450 system and the second-generation antipsychotics. *J Psychiatry Neurosci* 2003; **28**:99–112.
12. Johansson I, Lundqvist E, Bertilsson L, Dahl ML, Sjoqvist F, Ingelman-Sundberg M, Inherited amplification of an active gene in the cytochrome P450 CYP2D locus as a cause of ultrarapid metabolism of debrisoquine. *Proc Natl Acad Sci USA* 1993; **90**:11825–11829.
13. Berecz R, LLerena A, de la Rubia A et al, Relationship between risperidone and 9-hydroxy-risperidone plasma concentrations and CYP2D6 enzyme activity in psychiatric patients *Pharmacopsychiatry* 2002; **35**:231–234.
14. Bork JA, Rogers T, Wedlund PJ, de Leon J, A pilot study on risperidone metabolism: the role of cytochromes P450 2D6 and 3A. *J Clin Psychiatry* 1999; **60**:469–476.
15. Ozdemir V, Kalow W, Posner P et al, CYP1A2 activity as measured by a caffeine test predicts clozapine and active metabolite steady-state concentration in patients with schizophrenia. *J Clin Psychopharmacol* 2001; **21**:398–407.
16. Bender S, Eap CB, Very high cytochrome P4501A2 activity and nonresponse to clozapine. *Arch Gen Psychiatry* 1998; **55**:1048–1050.
17. Ozdemir V, Kalow W, Okey AB et al, Treatment-resistance to clozapine in association with ultrarapid CYP1A2 activity and the C→A polymorphism in intron 1 of the CYP1A2 gene: effect of grapefruit juice and low-dose fluvoxamine. *J Clin Psychopharmacol* 2001; **21**:603–607.
18. Arranz MJ, Dawson E, Shaikh S et al, Cytochrome P4502D6 genotype does not determine response to clozapine. *Br J Clin Pharmacol* 1995; **39**:417–420.
19. McLeod HL, Siva C, The thiopurine S-methyltransferase gene locus – implications for clinical pharmacogenomics. [Review] [54 refs]. *Pharmacogenomics* 2002; **3**:89–98.

20. Pompeo F, Brooke E, Kawamura A, Mushtaq A, Sim E, The pharmacogenetics of NAT: structural aspects. [Review] [101 refs]. *Pharmacogenomics*. 2002; 3:19–30.
21. Basile VS, Ozdemir V, Masellis M et al, A functional polymorphism of the cytochrome P450 1A2 (CYP1A2) gene: association with tardive dyskinesia in schizophrenia. *Mol Psychiatry*, 2000; 5:410–417.
22. Ellingrod VL, Schultz SK, Arndt S, Association between cytochrome P4502D6 (CYP2D6) genotype, antipsychotic exposure, and abnormal involuntary movement scale (AIMS) score. *Psychiatr Genet* 2000; 10:9–11.
23. Busatto GF, Kerwin RW, Perspectives on the role of serotonergic mechanisms in the pharmacology of schizophrenia. *J Psychopharmacol* 1997; 11:3–12.
24. Schmidt AW, Lebel LA, Howard HR Jr, Zorn SH, Ziprasidone: a novel antipsychotic agent with a unique human receptor binding profile. *Eur J Pharmacol* 2001; 425:197–201.
25. Wong AH, Buckle CE, Van Tol HH, Polymorphisms in dopamine receptors: what do they tell us? *Eur J Pharmacol* 2000; 410:183–203.
26. Kohn Y, Ebstein RP, Heresco-Levy U et al, Dopamine D4 receptor gene polymorphisms: relation to ethnicity, no association with schizophrenia and response to clozapine in Israeli subjects. *Eur Neuropsychopharmacol* 1997; 7:39–43.
27. Rietschel M, Naber D, Oberlander H et al, Efficacy and side-effects of clozapine: testing for association with allelic variation in the dopamine D4 receptor gene. *Neuropsychopharmacology* 1996; 15:491–496.
28. Shaikh S, Collier DA, Sham P et al, Analysis of clozapine response and polymorphisms of the dopamine D4 receptor gene (DRD4) in schizophrenic patients. *Am J Med Genet* 1995; 60:541–545.
29. Suzuki A, Kondo T, Otani K et al, Association of the TaqI A polymorphism of the dopamine D(2) receptor gene with predisposition to neuroleptic malignant syndrome. *Am J Psychiatry* 2001; 158:1714–1716.
30. Arinami T, Gao M, Hamaguchi H, Toru M, A functional polymorphism in the promoter region of the dopamine D2 receptor gene is associated with schizophrenia. *Hum Mol Genet* 1997; 6:577–582.
31. Ohara K, Nagai M, Tani K, Nakamura Y, Ino A, Ohara K, Functional polymorphism of -141C Ins/Del in the dopamine D2 receptor gene promoter and schizophrenia. *Psychiatry Res* 1998; 81:117–123.
32. Shaikh S, Collier DA, Sham PC et al, Allelic association between a Ser-9-Gly polymorphism in the dopamine D3 receptor gene and schizophrenia. *Hum Genet* 1996; 97:714–719.
33. Scharfetter J, Chaudhry HR, Hornik K et al, Dopamine D3 receptor gene polymorphism and response to clozapine in schizophrenic Pakistani patients. *Eur Neuropsychopharmacol* 1996; 10:17–20.
34. Malhotra AK, Goldman D, Buchanan RW et al, The dopamine D3 receptor (DRD3) Ser9Gly polymorphism and schizophrenia: a haplotype relative risk study and association with clozapine response. *Mol Psychiatry* 1998; 3:72–75.
35. Staddon S, Arranz MJ, Mancama D, Mata I, Kerwin RW, Clinical applications of pharmacogenetics in psychiatry. *Psychopharmacology (Berl)* 2002; 162:18–23.
36. Ishiguro H, Okuyama Y, Toru M, Arinami T, Mutation and association analysis of the 5' region of the dopamine D3 receptor gene in schizophrenia patients: identification of the Ala38Thr polymorphism and suggested association between DRD3 haplotypes and schizophrenia. *Mol Psychiatry* 2000; 5:433–438.
37. Williams J, Spurlock G, Holmans P et al, A meta-analysis and transmission disequilibrium study of association between the dopamine D3 receptor gene and schizophrenia. *Mol Psychiatry* 1998; 3:141–149.
38. Basile VS, Masellis M, Badri F et al, Association of the MscI polymorphism of the

dopamine D3 receptor gene with tardive dyskinesia in schizophrenia. *Neuropsychopharmacology* 1999; **21**:17–27.

39. Lerer B, Segman RH, Fangerau H et al, Pharmacogenetics of tardive dyskinesia: combined analysis of 780 patients supports association with dopamine D3 receptor gene Ser9Gly polymorphism. *Neuropsychopharmacology* 2002; **27**:105–119.

40. Woo SI, Kim JW, Rha E et al, Association of the Ser9Gly polymorphism in the dopamine D3 receptor gene with tardive dyskinesia in Korean schizophrenics. *Psychiatry Clin Neurosci* 2002; **56**:469–474.

41. Arranz M, Collier D, Sodhi M et al, Association between clozapine response and allelic variation in 5-HT2A receptor gene. *Lancet* 1995; **346**:281–282.

42. Malhotra AK, Goldman D, Ozaki N, Breier A, Buchanan R, Pickar D, Lack of association between polymorphisms in the 5-HT2A receptor gene and the antipsychotic response to clozapine. *Am J Psychiatry* 1996; **153**:1092–1094.

43. Masellis M, Basile V, Meltzer HY et al, Serotonin subtype 2 receptor genes and clinical response to clozapine in schizophrenia patients. *Neuropsychopharmacology* 1998; **19**:123–132.

44. Nothen MM, Rietschel M, Erdmann J et al, Genetic variation of the 5-HT2A receptor and response to clozapine. *Lancet* 1995; **346**:908–909.

45. Arranz MJ, Munro J, Sham P et al, Meta-analysis of studies on genetic variation in 5-HT2A receptors and clozapine response. *Schizophr Res* 1998; **32**:93–99.

46. Lane H-Y, Chang Y-C, Chiu C-C, Chen M-L, Hsieh M-H, Chang W-H, Association of risperidone treatment response with a polymorphism in the $5-HT_{2A}$ receptor gene. *Am J Psychiatry* 2002; **159**:1593–1595.

47. Arranz MJ, Collier DA, Munro J et al, Analysis of a structural polymorphism in the 5-HT2A receptor and clinical response to clozapine, *Neurosci Lett* 1996; **217**:177–178.

48. Sodhi MS, Arranz MJ, Curtis D et al, Association between clozapine response and allelic variation in the 5-HT2C receptor gene. *Neuroreport* 1995; **7**:169–172.

49. Rietschel M, Naber D, Fimmers R, Moller HJ, Propping P, Nothen MM, Efficacy and side-effects of clozapine not associated with variation in the 5-HT2C receptor. *Neuroreport* 1997; **8**:1999–2003.

50. Yu YW, Tsai SJ, Lin CH, Hsu CP, Yang KH, Hong CJ, Serotonin-6 receptor variant (C267T) and clinical response to clozapine. *Neuroreport* 1999; **10**:1231–1233.

51. Leibowitz SF, Alexander JT, Hypothalamic serotonin in control of eating behavior, meal size, and body weight. *Biol Psychiatry* 1998; **44**:851–864.

52. Basile VS, Masellis M, McIntyre RS et al, Genetic dissection of atypical antipsychotic-induced weight gain: novel preliminary data on the pharmacogenetic puzzle. [Review] [193 refs] *J Clin Psychiatry* 2001; **62(Suppl)**:66.

53. Hong CJ, Lin CH, Yu YW, Yang KH, Tsai SJ, Genetic variants of the serotonin system and weight change during clozapine treatment. *Pharmacogenetics* 2001; **11**:265–268.

54. Reynolds GP, Zhang ZJ, Zhang XB, Association of antipsychotic drug-induced weight gain with a 5-HT2C receptor gene polymorphism. *Lancet* 2000: **359**:2086–2087.

55. Zhang Z, Zhang X, Yao Z et al, [Association of antipsychotic agent-induced weight gain with a polymorphism of the promotor region of the 5-HT2C receptor gene]. *Zhonghua Yi Xue Za Zhi* 2002; **82**:1097–1101.

56. Bono M, Cases A, Oriola J, Calls J, Torras A, Rivera F, Polymorphisms of the human alpha 2A-adrenergic receptor gene in a Catalan population: description of a new polymorphism in the promoter region. *Gene Geogr* 1996; **10**:151–159.

57. Lario S, Calls J, Cases A, Oriola J, Torras A, Rivera F, MspI identifies a biallelic polymorphism in the promoter region of the alpha 2A-adrenergic receptor gene. *Clin Genet* 1997; **51**:129–130.

58. Shibata K, Hirasawa A, Moriyama N, Kawabe K, Oawa S, Tsujimoto G, Alpha (1a)-adrenoceptor polymorphisms: Pharmacological characterization and association with benign prostatic hypertrophy. *Br J Pharmacol* 1997; **118**:1403–1408.

59. Bolonna AA, Arranz MJ, Munro J et al, No influence of adrenergic receptor polymorphisms on schizophrenia and antipsychotic response. *Neurosci Lett* 2000; **280**:65–68.

60. Mancama D, Arranz MJ, Munro J et al, Investigation of promoter variants of the histamine 1 and 2 receptors in schizophrenia and clozapine response. *Neurosci Lett* 2002; **333**:207–211.

61. Schumacher J, Schulze TG, Wienker TF, Rietschel M, Nothen MM, Pharmacogenetics of the clozapine response. *Lancet* 2000; **356**:506–507.

62. Jibson MD, Tandon R, New atypical antipsychotic medications. *J Psychiatr Res* 1998; **32**:215–228.

63. Gray JW, Collins C, Genome changes and gene expression in human solid tumors. *Carcinogenesis* 2000; **21**:443–452.

64. Van Der Pouw Kraan TC, Van Gaalen FA, Huizinga TW, Pieterman E, Breedveld FC, Verweij CL, Discovery of distinctive gene expression profiles in rheumatoid synovium using cDNA microarray technology: evidence for the existence of multiple pathways of tissue destruction and repair. *Genes Immun* 2003; **4**:187–196.

65. Zimmermann N, King NE, Laporte J et al, Dissection of experimental asthma with DNA microarray analysis identifies arginase in asthma pathogenesis. *J Clin Invest* 2003; **111**:1863–1874.

66. Debouck C, Goodfellow PN, DNA microarrays in drug discovery and development. *Nat Genet* 1999; **21(Suppl)**:48–50.

67. Hakak Y, Walker JR, Li C et al, Genome-wide expression analysis reveals dysregulation of myelination-related genes in chronic schizophrenia. *Proc Natl Acad Sci USA* 2001; **98**:4746–4751.

68. Middleton FA, Mirnics K, Pierri JN, Lewis DA, Levitt P, Gene expression profiling reveals alterations of specific metabolic pathways in schizophrenia. *J Neurosci* 2002; **22**:2718–2729.

69. Mirnics K, Middleton FA, Marquez A, Lewis DA, Levitt P, Molecular characterization of schizophrenia viewed by microarray analysis of gene expression in prefrontal cortex. *Neuron* 2000; **28**:53–67.

70. Bunney WE, Bunney BG, Vawter MP et al, Microarray technology: a review of new strategies to discover candidate vulnerability genes in psychiatric disorders. *Am J Psychiatry* 2003; **160**:657–666.

71. Marcotte ER, Srivastava LK, Quirion R, DNA microarrays in neuropsychopharmacology. *Trends Pharmacol Sci* 2001; **22**:426–436.

72. Niculescu AB III, Segal DS, Kuczenski R, Barrett T, Hauger RL, Kelsoe JR, Identifying a series of candidate genes for mania and psychosis: a convergent functional genomics approach. *Physiol Genomics* 2000; **4**:83–91.

73. Toyooka K, Usui M, Washiyama K, Kumanishi T, Takahashi Y, Gene expression profiles in the brain from phencyclidine-treated mouse by using DNA microarray. *Ann NY Acad Sci* 2002; **965**:10–20.

74. Aerts J, Wetzels Y, Cohen N, Aerssens J, Data mining of public SNP databases for the selection of intragenic SNPs. *Hum Mutat* 2002; **20**:162–173.

75. Thorisson GA, Stein LD, The SNP Consortium website: past, present and future. *Nucleic Acids Res* 2003; **31**:124–127.

76. Smeraldi E, Zanardi R, Benedetti F, Di Bella D, Perez J, Catalano M, Polymorphism within the promoter of the serotonin transporter gene and antidepressant efficacy of fluvoxamine. [see comments]. *Mol Psychiatry* 1998; **3**:508–511.

77. Zanardi R, Benedetti F, Di Bella D, Catalano M, Smeraldi E, Efficacy of paroxetine

in depression is influenced by a functional polymorphism within the promoter of the serotonin transporter gene. *J Clin Psychopharmacol* 2000; **20**:105–107.

78. Kim DK, Lim SW, Lee S et al, Serotonin transporter gene polymorphism and anti-depressant response. *Neuroreport* 2000; **11**:215–219.

79. Yoshida K, Ito K, Sato K et al, Influence of the serotonin transporter gene-linked polymorphic region on the antidepressant response to fluvoxamine in Japanese depressed patients. *Prog Neuro-Psychopharmacol Biol Psychiatry* 2002; **26**:383–386.

80. Schafer M, Rujescu D, Giegling I et al, Association of short-term response to haloperidol treatment with a polymorphism in the dopamine D(2) receptor gene. *Am J Psychiatry* 2001; **158**:802–804.

81. Arranz MJ, Munro J, Birkett J et al, Pharmacogenetic prediction of clozapine response. *Lancet* 2000; **355**:1615–1616.

chapter 6

Can the social environment cause schizophrenia?

Lydia Krabbendam and Jim van Os

Few would contest the fact that mental states are influenced by experiences relating to the social environment. The question thus becomes: are the mental states that form part of the diagnosis of schizophrenia, defined according to DSM, ICD or any other system's criteria, somehow generated from within, in isolation from environmental experience?

Much depends on how one wishes to conceive of the schizophrenia phenotype. If schizophrenia was the result of a single, fully penetrant cause such as a single gene, the distribution of the disorder would be truly dichotomous, with a very small proportion of the population affected (Figure 6.1a). In this scenario, it would be hard to argue that most of the incidence could be attributed to factors in the social environment alone. However, it is very unlikely that schizophrenia is caused by a single factor. A multifactorial aetiology, similar to that seen in other chronic diseases such as diabetes and cardiovascular disease, is much more likely.[1] Any disease that is subject to multiple causal influences is likely to exist in nature as a quantitative trait, with less severe, non-pathologic manifestations of the phenotype lying on a continuum from normal experiences to disorder. If there are, for example, five or more different causal factors underlying psychosis, the observed distribution of the trait is highly dependent on the degree to which these causes interact, their prevalence, and the degree to which their effect sizes differ. If the effect of each of the five causes was moderate, not hugely different in magnitude, and contributed additively to the risk function and independently of each other, it could be shown statistically that psychosis would exist in nature as a normal distribution of traits (Figure 6.1b). If the

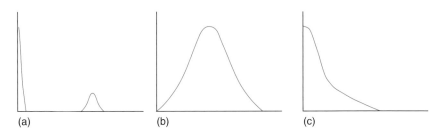

Figure 6.1 *Possible degrees of continuity of psychosis distributions. In (a) there is a clear bimodal distribution, with the great majority of the population having negligible values of the psychosis trait, whereas a very small proportion has extremely high values. In (b) there is a continuous and normal distribution of psychotic traits in the general population, much as one would expect of, for example, weight or blood pressure. In (c) there is a continuous but only half-normal distribution, with the majority of the population having very low values, but also a significant proportion with non-zero values.*

five causes both contributed independently and also co-participated to a degree, the distribution of the psychosis trait would lie somewhere between that of the dichotomous one in Figure 6.1a and the continuous one in Figure 6.1b (Figure 6.1c), depending on the degree of independent additive action and co-participation of the causes. In the case of large differences in effect size, with one or two very rare but extremely potent causes overshadowing the effect of more prevalent but weak causes, the appearance of the distribution would also be less continuous and more quasi-continuous. It can be surmised that the 'real' distribution of psychosis most likely lies somewhere between the dichotomous one in Figure 6.1a and the continuous one in Figure 6.1b, depending on the degree of interaction between the different causes and differences in their effect size.

Population variation argument

Continuity between the lesser psychotic states and clinical disorder would imply that risk factors that have been associated with the clinical disorder are also associated with the community level of psychotic symptoms. One way to study environmental risk factors is to compare populations with different mean levels of exposure and associate these with differences in the population levels of psychosis. This approach of showing between-population variation has been among the most successful to suggest a causal role of the social environment in schizophrenia. For example, incidence rates of schizophrenia vary widely, within the same country, between urban and rural populations,[2,3] and between majority and minority populations.[4,5] The question then becomes whether the established risk factors for schizophrenia also affect the occurrence of non-clinical psychosis-like experiences, in addition to occurrence of full-blown schizophrenic disorders. If, for example, the rate of some rare psychotic disorder is higher in population A than in population B, whereas their levels of more prevalent psychotic symptoms are the same, a likely explanation is that (i) some rare cause of a rare disorder is more prevalent in population A and (ii) psychosis-like experiences in the population are qualitatively distinct from the disorder. Thus, populations A and B are essentially similar, except for the distribution of some rare cause affecting a few individuals. There is variation within populations. If however, not only the rate of disorder, but also the rate of symptoms, are higher in population A than in population B, a likely explanation would be that (i) the population level of vulnerability differs between population A and population B and (ii) the psychosis-like experiences are, at least in part, on a quantitative continuum with the disorder.

Urbanicity and psychosis

Predictable differences in rates of psychotic disorder across different levels of urbanicity have been used to examine the population variation argument.[6] The hypothesis proposed was that the mean level of symptoms would increase with the rate of disorder across increasingly urbanized areas. In addition, it was hypothesized that the association between symptoms and disorder would be constant across the populations in the different strata, suggesting variation of susceptibility between populations rather than within populations. A random sample of 7076 men and women aged 18–64 years were interviewed by trained lay interviewers with the Composite International Diagnostic Interview (CIDI)[6] (the Dutch NEMESIS Study). Around half of those with evidence of psychosis according to the CIDI were additionally interviewed by clinicians. Subsequently, associations between a five-level urbanicity rating and (i) any DSM-III-R diagnosis of psychotic disorder (sample prevalence 1.5%), (ii) any rating of hallucinations and/or delusions (sample prevalence 4.2%) and (iii) any rating of psychotic or psychosis-like symptoms (sample prevalence 17.5%) were investigated. The results showed that level of urbanicity was not only associated with DSM-III-R psychotic disorder (adjusted odds ratio (OR) over five levels = 1.47, 95% confidence intervals (CI): 1.25 to 1.72), but also, independently, with any rating of delusion and/or hallucination (adjusted OR = 1.28, 95% CI 1.17 to 1.40 – clinician-assessed psychotic symptoms only: OR = 1.30, 95% CI 1.03 to 1.64), and any rating of psychosis-like symptom (adjusted OR = 1.18, 95% CI 1.13 to 1.24). Ratings of both lay interviewer and clinician-rated psychotic symptoms were strongly and independently associated with psychotic disorder, regardless of the level of urbanization. These findings suggest that the increased prevalence of psychotic disorder should be interpreted in light of increased levels of 'psychosis proneness' in urban populations. Since the association between symptoms and disorder did not differ as a function of urbanicity, the implication is, first, that susceptibility to psychotic disorder varies between populations and can be demonstrated by comparing rates of psychosis-like experiences, and second, that the psychosis-like experiences are on a quantitative continuum with the disorder.

Ethnicity and discrimination

Ethnic minority status is another source of variance between populations. Migrant groups with high rates of schizophrenia, such as African-Caribbean people living in the UK,[4,5] also have higher rates of psychosis-like phenomena.[8,9] These minority populations are not or are much less at risk in situations where they become majority populations,[10,11] indicating that genes alone cannot explain the findings. A recent study demonstrated that as the proportion of non-white ethnic minorities in a given neighbourhood decreases, the rate of incidence of schizophrenia increases.[12] This suggests an alternative mechanism, namely decreased exposure to, or increased protection from, racial discrimination in areas with relatively high proportions of ethnic minorities.

The effect of discrimination on the development of psychotic symptoms in the Dutch NEMESIS cohort was investigated prospectively.[13] At baseline, perceived discrimination on the basis of age, sex, handicap, appearance, skin colour or ethnicity and sexual orientation was assessed. The main outcome was onset of psychotic symptoms (delusions and hallucinations) at the 3-year follow-up. Delusional ideation was defined as a rating >1 for the Brief Psychiatric Rating Scale (BPRS) item 'unusual thought content', presence of hallucinations as a rating >1 for the BPRS item 'hallucinations'. The risk set consisted of individuals with no history of psychosis (n = 4076). This skewed the sample towards individuals with true first-ever occurrence of psychotic experiences at the follow-up and decreased bias due to the influence of baseline psychotic or psychosis-like symptoms on the reporting of discrimination (for example, individuals with paranoid symptoms may perceive, and report, more discrimination). The rate of delusional ideation was 0.5% (n = 19) in those who did not report discrimination, 0.9% (n = 4) in those who reported discrimination in one domain and 2.7% (n = 3) in those who reported discrimination in more than one domain (exact P = 0.027, OR = 2.1, 95% CI 1.2 to 3.8). This association remained after adjustment for possible confounders. No association was found between baseline discrimination and onset of hallucinatory experiences.

Perceived discrimination may induce delusional ideation and thus contribute to the high observed rates of psychotic disorder in exposed minority populations. There is growing evidence that cognitive attributions play a role in the onset of psychotic symptoms such as delusions by facilitating an understandably paranoid attributional style.[8,14]

Childhood trauma

Since these cognitive styles may develop early in life, it can be speculated that they are greatly influenced by adversities in early life.[15] We analysed data from the NEMESIS follow-up study in order to investigate the hypothesis that individuals from the general population who report childhood abuse are at increased risk of developing psychotic symptoms and psychotic disorder.[16] Again the risk set was restricted to those individuals with no previous lifetime presence of psychotic or psychosis-like symptoms in order to exclude the possibility that current psychotic beliefs would bias the way the abuse questionnaire was answered, and to be sure that the experience of abuse preceded the experience of psychotic symptoms. At baseline, using a semi-structured interview individuals were asked whether they had experienced any kind of emotional, physical, psychological or sexual abuse before age 16 years. The psychosis outcome was specified at three levels, two involving severity of positive symptoms of psychosis and one using additional clinical judgement of need for care: (i) any rating >1 on either BPRS item 'unusual thought content' or 'hallucinations' (BPRS any psychosis); (ii) any rating >3 on either 'unusual thought content' or 'hallucinations' (BPRS pathology-level psychosis); and (iii) need for care in relation to symptoms of psychosis was assessed by clinicians according to the Camberwell Assessment of Need.[17] Those who met criteria for BPRS pathology-level psychosis and clinician consensus on need for care, were defined as a case for treatment, hereafter referred to as 'need for care status'. The rate of BPRS any psychosis was 0.7% (n = 27) in those not exposed and 2.6% (n = 11) in those exposed to childhood abuse. For BPRS pathology-level psychosis, the rate was 0.1% (n = 4) in those not exposed and 1.4% (n = 6) in those who were exposed to childhood abuse. For those with need for care status, the rate was 0.1% (n = 3) for those not exposed and 0.9% (n = 4) for those exposed to childhood abuse. Childhood abuse was significantly associated with BPRS any psychosis (exact P = 0.001, OR = 3.6, 95% CI 1.8 to 7.2), with BPRS pathology-level psychosis (exact P = 0.000, OR = 13.0, 95%CI 3.7 to 46.3) and with need for care status (exact P = 0.003, OR = 11.5, 95%CI 2.6 to 51.6). After adjustment for possible confounders the risk decreased but remained large and significant for all three psychosis outcomes.

The results suggest that reported childhood abuse predicts psychotic disorder, but also psychotic and psychosis-like symptoms at lower levels of the continuum. Early adverse experiences such as social marginalization, childhood loss or severe childhood trauma, may create an enduring cognitive vulnerability, characterized by negative schematic models of the self and the world (e.g. beliefs about the self as vulnerable to threat, or about others as dangerous) that facilitate external attributions. This tendency to externally attribute events may lie beneath paranoid ideation.

Prenatal psychological exposures

The effects of psychological stress may already operate during prenatal development. Inconvenience of pregnancy and experience of stress during pregnancy have been associated with increased risk for schizophrenia.[18,19] We analysed data from a prospective cohort study of nearly 1000 adolescents and young adults in order to investigate the hypothesis that these psychological exposures would also be associated with higher levels of expression of non-clinical psychosis.[20] The Early Developmental Stages of Psychopathology (EDSP) study[21] is a longitudinal study of 963 adolescents aged 15–20 years and their parents. Adolescents were assessed by trained psychologists with the core psychosis sections on delusions and hallucinations of the Munich-Composite International Diagnostic Interview. Direct diagnostic interviews were conducted with the parents to obtain information about early development and familial psychopathology, including questions about perceived convenience of the pregnancy and stress during pregnancy. A total of 150 (15.6%) adolescents had ever had at least one psychotic experience, and 57 (5.9%) had had at least two psychotic experiences. Stress during pregnancy and inconvenience of pregnancy were associated with an increased risk of expression of psychosis in the adolescents (stress: OR 1.30, 95% CI 1.07 to 1.56; inconvenience: OR 1.79, 95% CI 1.16 to 2.75). Similar, but more enhanced, results were obtained with narrowly defined (at least two) psychotic experiences (stress: OR 1.65, 95% CI 1.28 to 2.12; inconvenience: OR 2.28, 95% CI 1.24 to 4.18). These effects remained after controlling for gender, socioeconomic status, as well as any psychiatric diagnosis and current level of depression and mania in the reporting parent.

The significance of these findings lies in the fact that prenatal risk factors may influence expression of psychosis outside the clinical phenotype. This suggests that the pathway from risk factors in early life to adult schizophrenia may involve an intermediary vulnerability state characterized by subtle but non-clinical psychotic experiences that may subsequently make the transition to clinical psychotic disorder, under the influence of other, more distal risk factors.[1,22,23]

Conclusion

The data presented in this chapter show that established proxy aetiological factors for schizophrenia such as urbanicity, discrimination, child abuse and prenatal exposures affect the occurrence of non-clinical psychosis-like experiences in addition to occurrence of full blown schizophrenic disorders. The environmental factors associated with these variables cause whole populations to have higher levels of non-clinical psychotic experiences, rather than causing a few individuals to develop a rare disorder (Figure 6.2). In other words, the psychosis phenotype appears to be a continuous function that varies with different levels of social environmental stresses. What is called schizophrenia may just be the extreme manifestation of this continuum. In conclusion, therefore, not only common sense but also research findings suggest that the mental states associated with schizophrenia are not the exception to the rule that psychological and environmental experiences go hand in hand.

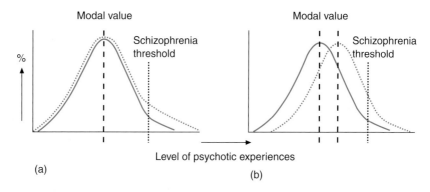

Figure 6.2 *Models explaining increased incidence rates of psychosis. Established proxy aetiological factors for schizophrenia cause a shift in the entire distribution of psychotic symptoms (b) rather than causing just a few individuals to develop a rare disorder (a).*

References

1. Johns LC, van Os J, The continuity of psychotic experiences in the general population. *Clin Psychol Rev* 2001; **21**:1125–1141.
2. Lewis G, David A, Andreasson S, Allebeck P, Schizophrenia and city life. *Lancet* 1992; **340**:137–140.
3. Marcelis M, Navarro Mateu F, Murray R, Selten JP, Van Os J, Urbanization and psychosis: a study of 1942–1978 birth cohorts in the Netherlands. *Psychol Med* 1998; **28**:871–879.
4. Harrison G, Owens D, Holton A, Neilson D, Boot D, A prospective study of severe mental disorder in Afro-Caribbean patients. *Psychol Med* 1988; **18**:643–657.
5. Sharpley MS, Hutchinson G, Murray RM, McKenzie K, Understanding the excess of psychosis among the African-Caribbean population in England: review of current hypotheses. *Br J Psychiatry* 2001; **178**:S60–68.
6. World Health Organization. Composite International Diagnostic Interview (CIDI); version 1.0 (RMW Smeets, PMAJ Dingemans, Trans.) Geneva: World Health Organization.
7. van Os J, Hanssen M, Bijl RV, Vollebergh W, Prevalence of psychotic disorder and community level of psychotic symptoms: an urban-rural comparison. *Arch Gen Psychiatry* 2001; **58**:663–668.
8. Sharpley MS, Peters ER, Ethnicity, class and schizotypy. *Soc Psychiatry Psychiatr Epidemiol* 1999; **34**:507–512.
9. Johns LC, Nazroo JY, Bebbington P, Kuipers E, Occurrence of hallucinatory experiences in a community sample and ethnic variations. *Br J Psychiatry* 2002; **180**:174–178.
10. Bhugra D, Hilwig M, Hossein B et al, First-contact incidence rates of schizophrenia in Trinidad and one-year follow-up. *Br J Psychiatry* 1996; **169**:587–592.
11. Hickling FW, Rodgers-Johnson P, The incidence of first contact schizophrenia in Jamaica. *Br J Psychiatry* 1995; **167**:193–196.
12. Boydell J, van Os J, McKenzie K et al, Incidence of schizophrenia in ethnic minorities in London: ecological study into interactions with environment. *BMJ* 2001; **323**:1336–1338.

13. Janssen I, Hanssen M, Bak M et al, Discrimination and delusional ideation. *Br J Psychiatry* 2003; **182**:71–76.
14. Bentall RP, Corcoran R, Howard R, Blackwood N, Kinderman P, Persecutory delusions: a review and theoretical integration. *Clin Psychol Rev* 2001; **21**:1143–1192.
15. Garety PA, Kuipers E, Fowler D, Freeman D, Bebbington PE, A cognitive model of the positive symptoms of psychosis. *Psychol Med* 2001; **31**:189–195.
16. Janssen I, Krabbendam L, Bak M et al, Childhood abuse as a risk factor for psychotic experiences. *Acta Psychiatr Scand* 2004; **109**:38–45.
17. Slade M, Phelan M, Thornicroft G, Parkman S, The Camberwell Assessment of Need (CAN): comparison of assessments by staff and patients of the needs of the severely mentally ill. *Soc Psychiatry Psychiatr Epidemiol* 1996; **31**:109–113.
18. Myhrman A, Rantakallio P, Isohanni M, Jones P, Partanen U, Unwantedness of a pregnancy and schizophrenia in the child. *Br J Psychiatry* 1996; **169**:637–640.
19. van Os J, Selten JP, Prenatal exposure to maternal stress and subsequent schizophrenia. The May 1940 invasion of The Netherlands. *Br J Psychiatry* 1998; **172**:324–326.
20. Spauwen J, Krabbendam L, Lieb R, Wittchen HU, van Os J, Sex differences in psychosis: normal or pathological? *Schizophr Res* 2003; **62**:45–49.
21. Lieb R, Wittchen HU, Hofler M, Fuetsch M, Stein MB, Merikangas KR, Parental psychopathology, parenting styles, and the risk of social phobia in offspring: a prospective-longitudinal community study. *Arch Gen Psychiatry* 2000; **57**:859–866.
22. Murray RM, Lewis SW, Is schizophrenia a neurodevelopmental disorder? *BMJ* (*Clin Res Ed*) 1988; **296**:63.
23. Jones PB, Rantakallio P, Hartikainen AL, Isohanni M, Sipila P, Schizophrenia as a long-term outcome of pregnancy, delivery, and perinatal complications: a 28-year follow-up of the 1966 north Finland general population birth cohort. *Am J Psychiatry* 1998; **155**:355–364.

chapter 7

The paradox of emotional dysfunction in 'non-affective' psychosis

Max Birchwood

Emotional dysfunction and schizophrenia have long been uncomfortable bedfellows. It was Bleuler who first argued that problems of affect lie at the heart of schizophrenia and that the symptoms we all focus on, the hallucinations and delusions, are merely 'accessory' and common to many forms of disorder. This view gave way to the now familiar distinction between affective and non-affective psychosis and to Jaspers' hierarchical approach to diagnosis wherein affective symptoms are 'trumped' by the presence of schizophrenia in terms of diagnosis and treatment. Yet emotional dysfunction is pervasive in non-affective psychosis! Sometimes (and unhelpfully) referred to as 'comorbidity', this includes: depression, usually accompanied by hopelessness and suicidal thinking; social anxiety, usually accompanied by social avoidance and problems forming relationships; and traumatic (post-traumatic stress disorder; PTSD) symptoms. There is also the distress (fear, anger, shame) attached to the experience of psychotic symptoms themselves. Emotional dysfunction, in common with the core symptoms and disabilities, develops rapidly and aggressively during the prodrome and early phase (Table 7.1).[1]

Following the first episode: over 50% report 'post-psychotic depression'[2] during a period which carries a high risk for suicide;[3] over a third report traumatic reactions sufficient to qualify for a diagnosis of PTSD, in particular, unwanted intrusions of images surrounding the first episode and its treatment;[4] and approaching 50% display a 'marked and persistent fear of social interaction', i.e. social anxiety disorder.[5] Perhaps more important for the person with psychosis is the problem of developing and maintaining

Table 7.1 Emotional dysfunction in first and multiple-episode psychosis

	Multiple episode (%)	*First episode (%)*
Depression	Up to 75 (40)	22–80 (50)
Suicidal ideation	40	50
Completed suicides	9–15	6?
Drug abuse	50	38
Alcohol abuse	10–58	24
Anxiety disorder	28–63	46
PTSD	51	35

PTSD, post-traumatic stress disorder.

intimate relationships: few people with psychosis will marry or have lasting relationships and many find themselves isolated and marginalized from social networks. Making clear diagnostic distinctions between these emotional disorders is not easy even in non-psychotic populations, where, for example, PTSD and depression overlap.[6]

It is tempting to characterize these emotional problems as simply part and parcel of psychosis (e.g. negative symptoms such as blunted or flattened emotion) and the loss of functioning which accompanies it (e.g. depressed Global Assessment of Functioning; GAF) and it is perhaps for this reason that the pathogenesis of these emotional difficulties is not understood and few effective treatments are available.[7] This is particularly important since the presence of these emotional disorders increases the probability of early relapse and their presence during the prodrome may act as risk factors for transition to psychosis.[8]

How are we to make sense of these disorders of emotion in an illness that is supposedly non-affective? I believe that in order to improve our understanding and to develop new treatments one needs to make a clear distinction between three core, but not mutually exclusive, pathways: emotional disorder that is *intrinsic* to the psychosis diathesis, a *psychological reaction* to it or the product of *disturbed developmental pathways*.

Emotional disorder as intrinsic to psychosis

The clearest example of an emotional disorder as intrinsic to psychosis is depression. The second generation of factor analytic studies of psychotic symptoms yields an additional dimension of depressive symptoms alongside the positive and negative dimensions. When orthogonality is not imposed on these factors, these dimensions co-vary within patient and community samples.[9] Depression is nearly always part of the first episode prodrome[10] that recedes with the positive symptoms.[2] The process underlying this link between positive symptoms, negative symptoms and depression is unknown but biological and psychological (see below) processes are plausible.

The therapeutic implications of this pathway to emotional disorder lie in the treatment of core psychotic symptoms.

Emotional disorder as a psychological reaction to psychosis

When considering emotional disorder as a psychological reaction, the emphasis is on psychosis, and the experience of psychotic symptoms, as a challenging or traumatic life event that requires adaptation by individuals and their families. Post-psychotic depression (PPD) is known to occur some months after recovery from the acute episode and has been shown by Birchwood et al to be predicted by how patients appraise the personal threat of this shattering life event: where the individual appraises psychosis as leading to *loss* of social goals, roles and status, as a source of *shame*, and from which escape is thwarted, i.e. *entrapment* by a supposed malignant disorder, this predicts the later emergence of PPD with hopelessness.[9] In this study, first episodes had a higher rate of PPD (over 50%), compared with multiple-episode patients (30%), linked to heightened awareness of the diagnosis and its implications in the aftermath of the first episode.

Where symptoms persist, depression has been traced to the *perceived* power of voices,[11] and of persecutory delusions,[12] and to the *subjective* experience of negative symptoms.[13] In general, the distress occasioned by persisting symptoms has been shown to operate through a 'psychological filter': those patients with more positive self-schema and personal resilience seem able to withstand the threat of voices or other persecutors.[11,12]

For example, in a series of studies it has been shown that the *relationship* with the voice in people who hear voices (one of subordination to a dominant power) is also manifest in the individual's social relationships, such that the individual feels subordinate and powerless in all interpersonal relationships. In a recent study of over 125 voice hearers,[30] a path analysis (covariance modelling) showed that these *social* appraisals were primary and appeared to underpin the dominant–subordinate relationship between the individual and their voice (Figure 7.1). This study, in keeping with previous ones, showed that over two-thirds of voice hearers were 'depressed'; however, it was not voice frequency or audibility that lay behind this, but these social appraisals of low social status and power. Such appraisals represent the 'psychological filter' which determines whether primary psychotic experiences are perceived as distressing and problematic.

With regard to traumatic reactions, evidence suggests that there is no link with the 'objective' trauma of psychosis, e.g. compulsory admission, as would be required for a DSM-IV diagnosis,[4,14] which has raised questions about the validity of the diagnosis. In non-psychotic PTSD, attention now focuses on the *perceived* threat of traumatic events and how people cope;[15] equally, in psychosis, patients may perceive themselves at risk of injury or death from supposed persecutors,[12] voices[11] or from others in a disturbed psychiatric ward, but its impact on trauma is as yet unknown. In other words, although individuals may not experience an actual threat of harm, they may, however, *perceive* such a threat, with traumatic consequences.

Turning to social anxiety, it is known that patients perceive themselves to be shamed and socially subordinated by others because of their psychosis

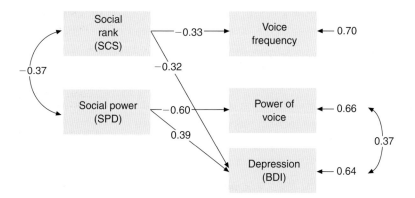

Figure 7.1 *Appraisals of social rank or position underlie appraisal of voices' power. Social rank and power primary ($\chi^2 = 1.2$, df = 3, P = 0.75). (Note: all parameter estimates statistically significant at P < 0.005.) BDI, Beck depression inventory; SCS, social comparison scale; SPD, social power differential scale.*

and patient status:[16] in non-psychotic social anxiety, patients fear criticism and humiliation in social encounters, which drives social avoidance.[17] It has been argued that a similar process, namely social shame and fear of discovery, may also underpin avoidance in psychosis.[11]

In a similar vein, the problems of fear and social avoidance in the context of active psychotic symptoms may be traced to the supposed threat posed by others: patients with persecutory delusions often deal with the perceived threat to their wellbeing through avoidance of high risk social encounters; in cognitive therapy this is one of a class of 'safety behaviours' which function to reduce threat.[12] Social disengagement can also be traced to the content of command hallucinations that can directly undermine trust in others.[18]

The therapeutic emphasis in this pathway focuses on patients' appraisals (beliefs, cognitions) of the threat posed by the diagnosis, by voices and by perceived social shame. The appraisal of loss is a key one in the genesis of depression,[19] whereas in PTSD, for example, it is the appraisal of *threat* which is important. Developmental experiences such as trauma predispose individuals to catastrophic appraisals of life events that act as a trigger for unipolar depression, and we may hypothesize that the same may also operate in psychosis (Figure 7.2).

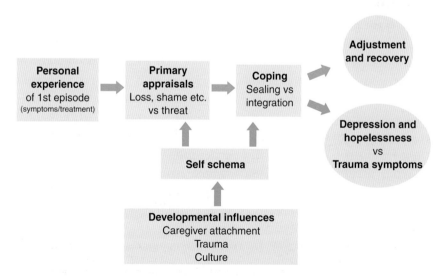

Figure 7.2 *Emotional dysfunction as a psychological reaction to psychosis.*

Disorders of emotion arising from developmental anomaly and trauma

Birth cohort and retrospective studies (e.g. Isohanni et al[20]) reveal that first episode psychosis is often preceded by social difficulty and emotional disorder as well as low level 'psychotic' experience stretching back into early adolescence.[21] These childhood antecedents of a developing psychosis will unfold in a social environment, and there is now considerable evidence that social factors influence morbidity and outcome of psychosis, for example, urban living (particularly deprivation), membership of marginalized social groups, the impact of migration and the (favourable) correlates of 'developing nation' status.[1] These unfolding antecedents of psychosis and the social risk factors will also affect 'normal' social and psychological development leading to low self-esteem, difficulty in establishing relationships, and susceptibility to stress. The science of 'developmental psychopathology'[21] shows that there exists continuity between adolescent and adult emotional disorder, including depression and risk of suicide, which occurs in a dimensional and not a categorical way, influenced by social and familial context.[22] *Dis*continuity between adolescent and adult emotional functioning is also possible; for example, Andrews and Brown[23] show that positive life events in late adolescence can help to restore a disturbed developmental trajectory back to within normal limits. The domains of emotional functioning in adolescence also interact; for example, social anxiety increases the developmental risk of adolescent depression.[24]

It is well established that developmental trauma and difficulty can act as risk factors for adult emotional disorder; for example, childhood abuse or neglect and problems of parental attachment can predispose to adult depression.[25] There is evidence of a high rate of traumatic histories in people with psychosis, including sexual trauma and emotional neglect, unwanted pregnancy and dysfunctional parental attachment (e.g. Greenfield et al[26]). These traumatic histories may also render patients prone to PPD and other emotional disorders: in PTSD, for example, traumatic responses to violent crime have been shown to be more likely in those with a history of childhood trauma who appraise the traumatic event as more personally threatening.[27]

In the cognitive framework, traumatic histories and developmental anomalies have been hypothesized to influence cognitive schema that govern the processing of self and social information. Such schema have been observed to be active in the emotional response to psychosis in the way in which the voice hearer appraises the interpersonal significance of the voice (i.e. of power and omnipotence)[11] and also in the distress and persistence of voices in young adolescents.[28]

In sum, this pathway to emotional disorder in first episode psychosis involves developmental disturbance triggered by an emerging psychosis, childhood trauma or both leading to (i) dysfunctional cognitive schema that affect adaptation to psychosis and its symptoms and (ii) adolescent emotional disorder that shows continuity into adulthood.

The therapeutic implications of this pathway lie in the focus on disturbances in 'normal' developmental processes in adolescence and their continuity with emerging psychopathology with a particular therapeutic focus on dysfunctional schema of self and others.

Conclusion

Distress from psychotic experience and the disorders of emotion in first episode psychosis may arise from three overlapping processes, including those which are intrinsic to psychosis, those which are a psychological reaction to psychosis and patienthood and those arising from anomalies of childhood and adolescent development, triggered by an emerging psychosis, childhood trauma or both. The application of cognitive behavioural therapy (CBT) in psychosis focuses on reducing psychotic symptoms as a means of alleviating the distress and emotional problems they give rise to – a quasi neuroleptic. The outcomes of CBT for psychosis have not shown consistent evidence for their impact on depression or other emotional dysfunctions; the same can be said for the neuroleptics. This analysis suggests a complementary and perhaps more fruitful focus on the concomitant emotional dysfunctions and their developmental and psychological origins. This will require the adaptation of tried and tested CBT for non-psychotic emotional disorder but also, crucially, a recognition that the powerful evidence for biological processes in psychosis sits comfortably side by side with developmental psychology and psychopathology; and for services, there will be much to gain from a cross-fertilization of approaches between Child and Adolescent Mental Health Services (CAMHS), youth and adult services in the management of first episode psychosis.

Implications for treatment

The core proposition outlined in this chapter is that distress and the emotional dysfunctions arising from psychosis can emerge from pathways that are not always driven by positive symptoms or primary psychotic experience. It is not surprising, therefore, that the mainstay of treatment, the neuroleptic, which aims to eliminate the positive symptoms, is neither necessary nor sufficient to eliminate distress and emotional dysfunction; for example, depression and suicide often occur following recovery from acute psychosis. Even cognitive therapy for psychosis, which focuses on delusional beliefs, including beliefs about voices, will not address all of these pathways and consequently fails to treat emotional dysfunction, particularly depression.[29] Moreover, it can be argued that it may be possible to reduce distress and behaviour arising from psychosis, without changing the core psychotic experience. For example, in recent work with command hallucinations[18] it was demonstrated that by focusing on the voice hearer's appraisal of the power and omnipotence of voices, this itself reduced depression and despair and compliance with voices' commands, but did not lead to a decrease in the frequency of hallucinations per se. It is my belief that the time has come to shift attention from CBT as a 'quasi-neuroleptic', to CBT as a therapy to relieve distress associated with psychotic experience and the 'comorbid' emotional dysfunctions, which should become the primary outcomes in CBT trials. CBT has, I believe, a *distinctive* role to play in relieving distress, which is more in keeping with its natural roots in the understanding and treatment of emotional dysfunction.

Acknowledgements

The author is grateful to Prof Glynn Harrison, Dr Paul Patterson and Dr Chris Jackson for helpful comments on an earlier version of this chapter.

References

1. Harrison G, Hopper K, Craig T et al, Recovery from psychotic illness: a 15- and 25-year international follow-up study. *Br J Psychiatry* 2001; **178**:506–517.
2. Birchwood M, Meaden A, Trower P, The power and omnipotence of voices: subordination and entrapment by voices and significant others. *Psychol Med* 2000; 30:337–344.
3. Westermeyer JF, Harrow M, Marengo JT, Risk for suicide in schizophrenia and other psychotic and nonpsychotic disorders. *J Nerv Ment Dis* 1991; **179**:259–266.

4. McGorry P, Chanen A, McCarthy E et al, Posttraumatic stress disorder following recent-onset psychosis: an unrecognized postpsychotic syndrome. *J Nerv Mental Dis* 1991; **179**:253–258.
5. Cosoff SJ, Hafner RJ, The prevalence of comorbid anxiety in schizophrenia, schizoaffective disorder and bipolar disorder. *Aust NZ J Psychiatry* 1998; **32**:67–72.
6. Bleich A, Koslowsky M, Dolev A et al, Post-traumatic stress disorder and depression – an analysis of comorbidity. *Br J Pschiatry* 2000; **170**:479–482.
7. Whitehead CMA, Cardno G Lewis, Antidepressants for the treatment of depression in people with schizophrenia: a systematic review. *Psychol Med* 33:589–599.
8. Strakowski SM, Keck PE Jr, McElroy SL et al, Chronology of comorbid and principal syndromes in first-episode psychosis. *Compr Psychiatry* 1995; **36**:106–112.
9. Stefanis NC, Hanssen M, Smirnis NK et al, Evidence that three dimensions of psychosis have a distribution in the general population. *Psychol Med* 2002; 32:347–358.
10. Jackson HJ, McGorry P, McKenzie D, The reliability of DSM-III prodromal symptoms in first episode psychotic patients. *Acta Psychiatr Scand* 1994; **90**:375–378.
11. Birchwood M, Iqbal Z, Chadwick P et al, Cognitive approach to depression and suicidal thinking in psychosis. I. Ontogeny of post-psychotic depression. *Br J Psychiatry* 2000; **177**:516–521.
12. Freeman D, Garety PA, Kuipers E, Persecutory delusions: developing the understanding of belief maintenance and emotional distress. *Psychol Med* 2001; 31:1293–1306.
13. Liddle PF, Barnes TRE, Curson DA et al, Depression and the experience of psychological deficits in schizophrenia. *Acta Psychiatr Scand* 1993; **88**:243–247.
14. Priebe S, Broker M, Gunkel S, Involuntary admission and posttraumatic stress disorder symptoms in schizophrenia patients. *Compr Psychiatry* 1998; **39**:220–224.
15. Ehlers A, Clark DM, A cognitive model of posttraumatic stress disorder. *Behav Res Ther* 2000; **38**:319–345.
16. Haghighat R, A unitary theory of stigmatisation – pursuit of self-interest and routes to destigmatisation. *Br J Psychiatry* 2001; **178**:207–215.
17. Clark DM, A cognitive perspective on social phobia. In: Crozier R, Alden LE (eds), *Handbook of Social Anxiety: concepts relating to the self and shyness.* Wiley: Chichester, 2001.
18. Trower P, Birchwood M, Meaden A, Byrne S, Nelson A. Cognitive therapy for command hallucinations: results of a randomised controlled trial. *Br J Psychiatry* (In Press).
19. Brown GW, Harris TO, Hepworth C. Loss, humilation and entrapment among women developing depression – a patient and nonpatient comparison. *Psychol Med* 1995; **25**:7–21.
20. Isohanni I, Jarvelin MR, Nieminen P et al, School performance as a predictor of psychiatric hospitalization in adult life. A 28-year follow-up in the Northern Finland 1966 Birth Cohort. *Psychol Med* 1998; **28**:967–974.
21. Poulton R, Caspi A, Moffitt TE et al, Children's self-reported psychotic symptoms and adult schizophreniform disorder – a 15-year longitudinal study. *Arch Gen Psychiatry* 2000; **57**:1053–1058.
21. Rutter M, Risks and outcomes in developmental psychopathology. *Br J Psychiatry* 2000; **177**:569–569.
22. Fombonne E, Wostear G, Cooper V et al, The Maudsley long-term follow-up of child and adolescent depression. 1. Psychiatric outcomes in adulthood. *Br J Psychiatry* 2001; **179**:210–217.
23. Andrews B, Brown GW, Stability and change in low self-esteem – the role of psychosocial factors. *Psychol Med* 1995; **25**:23–31.

24. Stein MB, Fuetsch M, Muller N et al, Social anxiety disorder and the risk of depression: a prospective community study of adolescents and young adults. *Arch Gen Psychiatry* 2001; **58**:251–256.

25. Bifulco A, Brown GW, Moran P et al, Predicting depression in women: the role of past and present vulnerability. *Psychol Med* 1998; **28**:39–50.

26. Greenfield SF, Strakowski SM, Tohen M et al, Childhood abuse in first-episode psychosis. *Br J Psychiatry* 1994; **164**:831–834.

27. Andrews B, Brewin CR, Rose S et al, Predicting PTSD symptoms in victims of violent crime: the role of shame, anger, and childhood abuse. *J Abnorm Psychol* 2000; **109**:69–73.

28. Escher S, Romme M, Buiks A, Delespaul P, van Os J, Independent course of childhood auditory hallucinations: a sequential 3-year follow up study. *Br J Psychiatry* 2002; **43**:S10–18.

29. Birchwood R, Spencer E, Indications and planning of psychotherapies for schizophrenia. In: Mario M, Sartorius N (eds), *WPA Series in Evidence & Experience in Psychiatry*. John Wiley & Sons: Chichester, 2003.

30. Birchwood M, Gilbert P, Gilbert J, Trower P, Meaden A, Murray J, Interpersonal and role-related schema influence the relationship with the dominant 'voice' in schizophrenia: a comparison of the three models. *Psychol Med* (in press).

chapter 8

Risk and protective factors

Glyn Lewis and Stan Zammit

Epidemiology is concerned, in part, with investigating the causes of disease in human populations. In psychiatry, epidemiologists study the relationship between biological or psychological factors and mental illness in human populations. Epidemiology therefore is about understanding the biology of mental illness and informing the mechanisms that underlie mental illness.

One of the areas that has led to confusion between epidemiologists and investigators interested in the biology of schizophrenia is that at first sight we have quite different causal models of disease. Within epidemiology there is the acceptance that causal factors are neither necessary nor sufficient to cause disease. In other words someone with the presumed risk factor need not develop the disease and someone without the risk factor can also develop the disease. It is another way of explaining those elderly relatives who appear to have smoked all their lives without any obvious harm to their health. As a result the causal factors in epidemiological research tend to be called 'risk factors' in the sense that they increase the risk of developing disease. In contrast, most of the biological approaches towards under-standing causal mechanisms rely upon a much more mechanistic approach in which disease is inevitable, given various combinations of factors. Most biological approaches regard causes as sufficient, even if they are not necessary. Perhaps this view of the biological approach is somewhat extreme but it does reflect the difference in attitude towards cause between epidemi-ologists and biologists. For example, geneticists concerned with complex dis-eases are increasingly adopting a view of causation similar to that of epidemiologists.

The epidemiologist Rothman has suggested a way of reconciling these two apparently contradictory approaches.[1] Rothman has suggested that each disease is likely to show some heterogeneity in which a variety of different causal 'pie charts' can all lead to a common final pathway for a disease. Each of these individual pie charts would fit with a mechanistic biological model

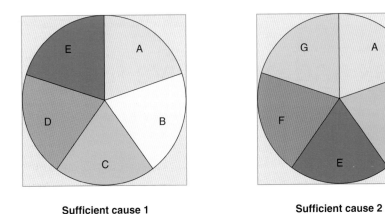

Sufficient cause 1   **Sufficient cause 2**

Figure 8.1 *Two sufficient causes for disease with overlapping causal factors.*

of disease in which everyone with all those factors would inevitably develop the disease. In that sense each pie chart is a 'sufficient cause'. For each disease there will be several sufficient causes in which different but overlapping combinations of factors are all required to explain the onset of disease (Figure 8.1). Within each pie chart there is a strict mechanistic causal relationship but in a study, each risk factor behaves as though it were neither necessary nor sufficient for the onset of a disease. For example, in Figure 8.1 factor B would neither be necessary nor sufficient for the occurrence of disease.

Epidemiology has therefore often led the way in understanding the relationship between biology and disease. There have been many circumstances when epidemiological observations have led on to areas of biological research. For example, research on cigarette smoking and lung cancer, cervical cancer and the human papillomavirus, oestrogens and breast cancer all began with an epidemiological observation.[2,3] John Snow was the founding father of epidemiology and also discovered the link between contaminated water and the clinical syndrome of cholera, many years before the cholera vibrio was discovered. This should provide encouragement for psychiatric epidemiologists who have to work in an area of great biological uncertainty and should also serve as a reminder for biologists to attend to epidemiological findings. One of the observations that led on to Snow's studies[4] was the low rate of incidence of cholera among the workers in the brewery in Broad Street, London, in the 1850s. We suppose one interpretation was that this resulted from the health benefits of drinking beer to the exclusion of almost any other liquids. However, John Snow concluded it resulted from avoiding drinking the contaminated water of the time.

The rest of this chapter will apply these general observations to schizophrenia concentrating on two areas: asphyxia at birth and smoking in young adulthood.

Asphyxia at birth

The literature on complications of birth and delivery and schizophrenia is large and rather contradictory.[5] Some of the earlier studies suffered from a number of quite important methodological limitations but there are now some recent studies that have adopted much more robust methods. Another limitation of much of the earlier research was that different aspects of birth and delivery complications were treated as though they were a single pathological process. For example, the presence or absence of obstetric complications has often been a composite item that might include problems around birth, caesarian sections or low birthweight. These various obstetric complications almost certainly reflect quite different pathological processes. It is clearly not sensible to lump all complications in together, because they are dealing with quite different biological mechanisms. In biological terms, it is probably possible to distinguish between two areas of birth and delivery complications. One mechanism might be some abnormality during fetal life, a chronic abnormality that affects growth and the developing brain. The other possible biological trauma might be a more acute delivery complication, such as asphyxia during birth, which would presumably have different consequences for the developing fetus and might damage different areas of the brain.

We carried out a case–control study with colleagues from Sweden, looking at cases from the Stockholm County Case Register, who were born in Stockholm County after about 1960.[6] The selected controls were born in the same area and still living in Stockholm during the period of risk for the cases. This selection procedure was a way of reducing the possibility of selection bias and to make sure that the case–control study was population-based. The notes for both cases and controls were extracted and midwives – unaware of case and control status – screened these for possible asphyxia. Then a paediatrician also blind to the case and control status examined the notes with possible asphyxia and indicated whether asphyxia was present to a sufficient degree to lead to a score of less than 7 on the Apgar scale at 5 minutes.

Before the study was started a number of features were selected that indicated a disorder during pregnancy that might affect fetal growth or development. These included birthweight, length, gestation, delay in gaining weight after birth and pre-eclampsia. We also decided on indicators of asphyxia around birth such as instrument delivery, low or high fetal heart rate, remaining in hospital after delivery and a long labour. However, these are very poor measures of birth asphyxia, especially under relatively modern obstetric practices. This study was undertaken in Sweden, which has some of the lowest rates of delivery complications in the world and very good neonatal survival. Our Paediatrician assessment of asphyxia should be a more robust measure. The results of the univariate analysis showed several factors were associated with schizophrenia, for example, low birthweight was associated with schizophrenia. The asphyxia measure and whether the child remained in hospital after birth, a possible sign of problems at birth, were also associated with schizophrenia in this analysis.

It is important to acknowledge that these obstetric and delivery variables are all associated with each other and so to understand possible causal mechanisms it is essential to adjust for the other obstetric variables. It is then possible that a clear-cut pattern might emerge. After adjustment, it was found that in the study sample asphyxia at birth was associated with an increased risk of schizophrenia (odds ratio 4.4, 95% CI 1.9 to 10.3) and this was independent of all the other factors that were measured and investigated including birthweight, gestation, pre-eclampsia and maternal history of psychosis. In other words, the association between these factors and schizophrenia in the univariate or unadjusted analysis could be explained because, for example, babies with low birthweight were also more likely to experience asphyxia around birth.

In conclusion, a strong association with birth asphyxia was found; this confounded the relationship with a number of other birth complications. In contrast with most other studies, the presence of asphyxia in this study was determined by paediatricians examining case notes and did not rely upon the routinely available data from databases. It is possible that this is a much more accurate way of establishing presence of asphyxia than by using routine data that might be of less quality. What might this result, if confirmed, mean from a biological perspective? It suggests a number of different lines of enquiry. For example, what areas of the brain are susceptible to anoxic damage around birth? What kind of protective mechanisms exist in neonates that reduce the possibility of anoxic damage? Is there individual, perhaps genetic variation in these protective mechanisms? If we understood more about the biology of asphyxia at birth and the impact on the brain, this could lead on to more accurately specified biological hypotheses and might also provide clues about what genes might be involved in the aetiology of schizophrenia.

Smoking and schizophrenia

People with schizophrenia are more likely to smoke cigarettes. This association has been observed in many case–control and cross-sectional studies. There is probably a two- to three-fold increase in smoking frequency in people with schizophrenia compared with the general population and maybe slightly less when compared with other psychiatric diagnoses. However, these data are all from people who already have schizophrenia. It has been suggested that people with schizophrenia might consume tobacco in order to 'self-medicate' and it might relieve some of the more negative symptoms of schizophrenia.[7] It is therefore possible that tobacco consumption might alter the risk of developing schizophrenia in otherwise well individuals.

We along with colleagues from the Karolinska Institute, Stockholm, examined this possibility using the Swedish conscript survey, which has data on tobacco use by 18–20-year-old men.[8] About 50 000 male conscripts were surveyed in 1969 or 1970. The survey included about 97% of the 18–20-year-old male population of Sweden at the time. Some people were excluded because of ill health before they got to the screening stage and 34 people were excluded because they had a psychotic illness at baseline, established following a screening procedure. The conscripts were followed-up using the Swedish National Register of In-patient Care, and this gives a record of inpatient admissions for schizophrenia between 1970 and 1996.

No association between cigarette smoking and schizophrenia was found in the unadjusted results. However, when other confounding variables were adjusted for, particularly low intelligence quotient (IQ) score and drug use, there appeared to be a protective effect of smoking cigarettes and this was significant ($P = 0.002$). This association was relatively strong and those smoking 20 or more cigarettes a day at age 18 years had half the risk of developing schizophrenia compared with non-smokers (hazard ratio 0.5, 95% CI 0.3 to 0.9). We stratified the analysis by the date of admission for schizophrenia to investigate whether any association was the result of a prodromal phase of schizophrenia, as a prodromal phase is expected to obscure the protective relation if people with schizophrenia smoke cigarettes to self-medicate. In the first 5 years after conscription, the possibly protective association with schizophrenia was less strong than in those people with schizophrenia presenting after 5 years.

First it is important to emphasize that any possible benefits of smoking cigarettes on reducing the risk of schizophrenia are overwhelmed by the considerable harm to physical health. We were initially surprised by our findings but there are a number of independent features that are consistent with this finding of a possible protective effect of schizophrenia. For example, there is a quite robust finding that people who smoke cigarettes have a reduced risk of Parkinson's disease.[9] This was first reported in the British Doctors' Cohort study by Richard Doll and Bradford Hill.[10] There are also a number of plausible mechanisms by which nicotine might influence the onset or course of schizophrenia. Nicotine increases frontal dopamine transmission[11] and this may be reduced in people with schizophrenia. There is also evidence of a neuroprotective effect of nicotine in animal models.[12] Nicotine may reverse some of the abnormalities in prepulse inhibition that have been observed in people with schizophrenia.

If nicotine does influence the onset of schizophrenia it leads on to studying other factors, including genetic polymorphisms, that might affect nicotinic transmission in the central nervous system. There is also some evidence of linkage between schizophrenia and the area on chromosone 15 in the region of the α_7 nicotinic receptor. The possible association between smoking and schizophrenia has no real public health importance but may help to understand some of the molecular processes that cause schizophrenia.

Conclusion

The epidemiological associations reported above give some possible clues about the biological basis of schizophrenia. Clearly, they need to be replicated in other places and in other samples. However, if these associations are robust, they provide a scientific lead for the investigation of related biological abnormalities in schizophrenia. For example, if nicotine is important in the aetiology of schizophrenia, then functional abnormalities in the nicotinic receptor, particularly the α_7 receptor, may also alter risk of schizophrenia. This might be particularly marked in those who are consuming nicotine. Likewise, if asphyxia is important, variation in the mechanisms that protect the neonatal brain from ischaemic damage would be likely to affect the incidence of schizophrenia. These are important clues concerning the biological basis of schizophrenia and merit further investigation. Epidemiologists and biologists need to work together if progress is to be made in understanding this important condition.

References

1. Rothman K, Greenland S, *Modern Epidemiology*. Lippincott, Williams & Wilkins: Philadelphia, 1998.
2. Munoz N, Bosch FX, HPV and cervical neoplasia: review of case–control and cohort studies. In: Munoz N et al (eds), *The Epidemiology of Cervical Cancer and Human Papillomavirus*. IARC: Lyon, 1992.
3. Miller AB, Bulbrook RD, UICC multidisciplinary project on breast cancer: the epidemiology, aetiology and prevention of breast cancer. *Int J Cancer* 1986; **37**:173–177.
4. Snow J, On the mode of communication of cholera. The Commonwealth Fund: New York, 1936.
5. Cannon M, Jones P, Murray R, Obstetric complications and schizophrenia: historical and meta-analytic review. *Am J Psychiatry* 2002; **159**:1080–1092.
6. Dalman C, Thomas HV, David A, Gentz J, Lewis G, Allebeck P, Signs of asphyxia at birth and risk of schizophrenia. *Br J Psychiatry* 2001; **179**:403–408.
7. Adler LE, Hoffer LD, Wiser A, Freedman R, Normalization of auditory physiology by cigarette smoking in schizophrenic patients. *Am J Psychiatry* 1993; **150**:1856–1861.
8. Zammitt S, Allebeck A, Dalman C, Lundberg I, Hemmingsson T, Lewis G, Investigating the association between cigarette smoking and schizophrenia using a cohort study. *Am J Psychiatry* 2003; **160**:2216–2221.
9. Ben-Shlomo Y, How far are we in understanding the cause of Parkinson's disease. *J Neurol Neurosurg Psychiatry* 1996; **61**:4–16.
10. Doll R, Peto R, Wheatley K, Gray R, Sutherland I, Mortality in relation to smoking: 40 years' observations on male British doctors. *BMJ* 1994; **309**:901–911.
11. Drew AE, Derbez AE, Werling LL, Nicotinic receptor-mediated regulation of dopamine transporter activity in rat prefrontal cortex. *Synapse* 2000; **38**:10–16.
12. Belluardo N, Mudo G, Blum M, Fuxe K, Central nicotinic receptors, neurotrophic factors and neuroprotection. *Behav Brain Res* 2000; **113**:21–34.

chapter 9

What is the relationship between methamphetamine and cannabis abuse and schizophrenia?

Robin M Murray, Chih-Ken Chen, Anton Grech, Louise Arseneault, Mary Cannon and Jolanta Zanelli

This chapter addresses the nature of the relationship between schizophrenia and two drugs, methamphetamine and cannabis, which are frequently consumed by people with psychosis in the Pacific countries and Europe, respectively.

Methamphetamine and schizophrenia

The fact that amphetamine and its derivatives can induce a schizophrenia-like profile has been known for almost half a century.[1] Figure 9.1 shows the distribution in 163 psychotic patients of many of the symptoms that we associate with schizophrenia: 85% had auditory hallucinations; about 71% had delusions of persecution and 63% had delusions of reference; 47% had visual hallucinations; 41% had delusions of thought reading; 28% had delusions of thought insertion; 26% had delusions of thought broadcasting; 23% had delusions of being controlled; and 27% had odd speech.[2] However, these patients were not diagnosed with schizophrenia but rather with methamphetamine psychosis. Methamphetamine abuse is common in the Far East, and there is currently an epidemic of methamphetamine psychosis in Japan, Thailand and Taiwan. It appears that methamphetamine abuse can induce a psychosis almost identical to the positive syndrome of schizophrenia.

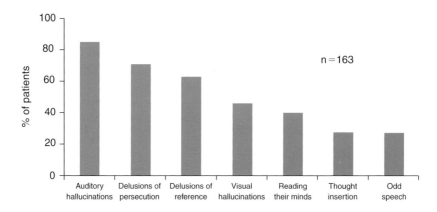

Figure 9.1 *Psychopathology of individuals with methamphetamine psychosis. (From Chen C-K et al. Psychol Med 2003.[2]*

Why do some methamphetamine abusers, however, continue to abuse the drug and never become psychotic, while others with a similar intake develop psychosis? To answer this question, we studied 121 regular abusers of methamphetamine who never developed psychosis, 140 who occasionally abused methamphetamine and never developed psychosis, 143 who had a psychosis that lasted less than 1 month and were abusing methamphetamine, and 20 methamphetamine abusers who had a psychosis that lasted more than 1 month.[2] Mothers were interviewed about childhood schizoid and schizotypal traits using a schedule described by Forester et al.[3] The results are illustrated in Figure 9.2. Individuals who developed psychosis, particularly a long-lasting episode, had shown more schizoid/schizotypal traits in childhood according to their mothers, while those who continued use of methamphetamine without developing psychosis had low rates of such traits in childhood. This finding suggests that those with childhood schizoid traits are at particular risk of developing psychosis, should they abuse methamphetamine.

Figure 9.3 shows the risk of schizophrenia in the first-degree relatives of the methamphetamine abusers. The relatives of those people who abused methamphetamine but who never became psychotic had a low morbid risk for schizophrenia; the relatives of those who became briefly psychotic showed a higher risk; and those who had a prolonged episode of psychosis showed the highest genetic loading. Thus methamphetamine abusers with familial/genetic predisposition are especially likely to develop psychosis.

These data suggest a graded predisposition to develop psychosis, with those individuals with familial predisposition and childhood schizoid/

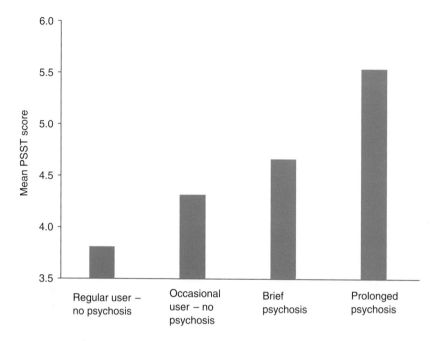

Figure 9.2 *Childhood schizoid/schizotypal traits in methamphetamine abusers divided by the presence and duration of psychosis. PSST, Premorbid Schizoid and Schizotypal Trait (Scale).*

schizotypal characteristics being at greatest risk of developing frank psychosis when exposed to repeated challenge with a drug known to increase synaptic dopamine. The same factors, which predispose to the occurrence of psychosis, predict its longevity.

Cannabis and schizophrenia

Another frequently used drug associated with psychosis is cannabis. Many studies show that psychotic patients use cannabis more than the general population.[4] In South London, it was found that patients with recent onset psychosis were approximately twice as likely to use cannabis than a comparable control population.[5] It is sometimes stated that psychotic patients take cannabis as an attempt to self-medicate either for anxiety or negative symptoms associated with the illness, or in order to counteract the side effects of antipsychotic medication. Should this be the case, and the drug be effective, then one would expect those psychotic patients who use cannabis to have a better outcome than those who do not use cannabis. However,

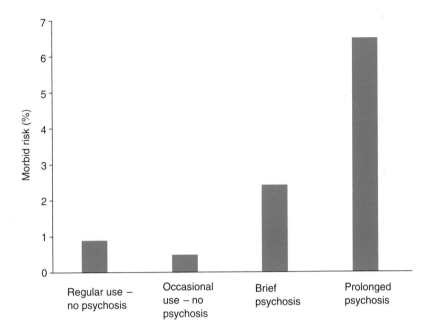

Figure 9.3 *Morbid risk of schizophrenia in relatives of 445 amphetamine abusers.*

when psychotic patients were followed up for 4 years, we found, as had others previously, that those individuals who continued to take cannabis had worse outcomes than those who did not; in particular, they were almost four times more likely to show positive psychotic symptoms at follow-up, three times more likely to have had a chronic course, and they were no less likely to show negative symptoms (Table 9.1).[5]

But does cannabis use increase the risk of psychosis as well as impairing the outcome of those already psychotic? The Swedish army study, by Andreasson et al, published in 1987 showed that admitting to have used cannabis at least 50 times by the age 18 years carried a six-fold increased risk of being diagnosed as schizophrenic over the next 15 years.[6] The findings of this single study had little influence, largely because no attempts were made at replication. However, several recent prospective studies have now been reported which have indeed replicated the findings.[7-9] Nevertheless, critics suggested that perhaps the initial cannabis consumption was a behavioural epiphenomenon of pre-schizophrenic individuals, i.e. those individuals at increased risk of psychosis are also at risk of using cannabis in adolescence.

This issue was addressed in a study of the Dunedin cohort of just over

Table 9.1 Effect of cannabis intake on outcome of psychosis at 4 years[5]

	Positive symptoms	Negative symptoms	Continuous course
No cannabis	1	1	1
Initially only	1.6	0.6	1.7
Both	3.7	1.1	2.8

1000 children in New Zealand.[10] The children were assessed in detail throughout childhood, and at age 26 years; 96% were interviewed using the Diagnostic Interview Schedule (DIS) for DSM IV.[11] Information about cannabis consumption at ages 15 and 18 years was evaluated in relation to risk of schizophreniform disorder at age 26 years. Those who were using cannabis at the age of 18 years were not more likely to develop schizophreniform disorder as adults. However, cannabis use by age 15 years carried a four-fold increased risk of schizophreniform psychosis in adulthood (Figure 9.4). Information on psychotic symptoms was collected prospectively when individuals were age 11 years. Poulton et al[12] demonstrated that children who answered positively to questions such as 'Do other people read your minds?', 'Have you ever heard messages sent to you through TV or radio?', 'Have you ever thought that people were following you or spying on you?' or 'Have you heard voices that other people can't hear?' were more likely to meet diagnostic criteria for schizophreniform disorder as adults. When the association between cannabis use at age 15 years and schizophreniform disorder was tested controlling for the presence of these psychotic symptoms at age 11 years, the odds ratio of schizophreniform disorder became non-significant although it remained raised at 3. In other words, individuals who had psychotic symptoms at age 11 years were particularly susceptible to develop psychosis later in life, but when this was taken into consideration, there was still an effect of early cannabis use on schizophrenia outcome.

Thus, it seems that consumption of cannabis not only makes those with established schizophrenia worse but it also can contribute to the onset of psychosis in the first place.

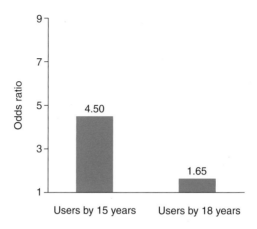

Figure 9.4 *Cannabis use in adolescence and schizophreniform disorder at age 26 years. (From Arseneault L et al.* BMJ *2002;* **325:***1212–1213.[11])*

References

1. Connell PH, *Amphetamine Psychosis*. Chapman Hall for the Institute of Psychiatry: Glasgow, 1958.
2. Chen C-K, Lin S-K, Sham P et al, Premorbid characteristics and comorbidity of methamphetamine users with and without psychosis. *Psychol Med* 2003; **33**:1407–1414.
3. Foerster A, Lewis G, Owen M et al, Premorbid adjustment and personality in psychosis. Effects of sex and diagnosis. *Br J Psychiatry* 1991; **58**:171–176.
4. Thornicroft G, Cannabis and psychosis. Is there epidemiological evidence for an association? [Erratum appears in *Br J Psychiatry* 1990; **157**:460] *Br J Psychiatry* 1990; **157**:25–33.
5. Grech A, Takei N, Murray R, Psychosis and cannabis use. *Schizophr Res* 1998; **29**:21.
6. Andreasson S, Allebeck P, Engstrom A, Rydberg U, Cannabis and schizophrenia. A longitudinal study of Swedish conscripts. *Lancet* 1987; **2**:1483–1486.
7. van Os J, Bak M, Hanssen M et al, Cannabis use and psychosis: a longitudinal population-based study. *Am J Epidemiol* 2002; **156**:319–327.
8. Zammit S, Allebeck P, Andreasson S et al, Self reported cannabis use as a risk factor for schizophrenia in Swedish conscripts of 1969: historical cohort study. *BMJ* 2002; **325**:1199–1201.
9. Fergusson DM, Horwood LJ, Swain-Campbell N, Cannabis use and psychosocial adjustment in adolescence and young adulthood. [Comment] *Addiction* 2002; **97**:1123–1135.
10. Moffitt TE, Caspi A, Rutter M, Silva PA, *Sex differences in antisocial behaviour: conduct disorder, delinquency, and violence in the Dunedin longitudinal study*. Cambridge University Press: Cambridge, 2001.
11. Arseneault L, Cannon M, Poulton R et al, Cannabis use in adolescence and risk for adult psychosis: longitudinal prospective study. *BMJ* 2002; **325**:1212–1213.
12. Poulton R, Caspi A, Moffitt TE et al. Children's self-reported psychotic symptoms and adult schizophreniform disorder: a 15-year longitudinal study. *Arch Gen Psychiatry* 2000; **57**:1053–1058.

chapter 10

Prediction of psychosis is necessary and possible

Frauke Schultze-Lutter

It has long been known that, in the vast majority of cases, schizophrenia is not a sudden event. In the Mannheim Age, Beginning, Course (ABC) study of 232 first admissions for first episode schizophrenia,[1] it was found that first hospitalization was preceded by a psychotic prephase in which psychotic symptoms had been present already for about 1 year and by an additional phase of an average of 5 years in which first negative or non-specific signs of a mental disorder had been present. This was true for about three-quarters of all patients. Furthermore, at the time of the first sign of mental illness, only insignificant differences were found between people who later developed schizophrenia (n = 57) and age, sex and place of residence matched controls (n = 57) with regard to different key roles for social role performance. However, at the time of first admission to hospital, this picture had changed and significant differences in social role performance were shown especially with regard to employment (t-test, $P < 0.10$), own income (t-test, $P < 0.01$) and stable partnership or marriage (t-test, $P < 0.001$). The onset of social disabilities that were assessed according to the Disability Assessment Schedule[2] on average clearly pre-dated the first admission and – by more than a year – even the onset of the first positive symptoms (Figure 10.1). Thus, social deficits that are often hard to treat after the first episode of schizophrenia seem to have developed already in the initial prodromal phase.

As a consequence of these findings and others, prediction of psychosis appears necessary, because:

- a prodromal phase is present in the majority of patients with first episode schizophrenia;[1]
- patients and their families suffer from symptoms and deficits occurring in this phase and they seek help for them;[3,4]

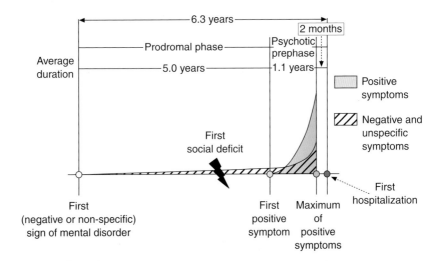

Figure 10.1 *Prephases of schizophrenia from first sign of mental disorder to first admission: results of the retrospective ABC study of 232 first admissions for schizophrenia. (Modified from Häfner H et al. In:* Risk and Protective Factors in Schizophrenia. *Darmstadt: Steinkopff, 2002.[1])*

- social deficits already seem to occur in the prodromal phase, prior to the first psychotic symptoms;[1]
- deterioration of functioning does not seem to be linear but tends to worsen for the first few years and then often reaches a plateau;[5] and
- the duration of untreated psychosis seems to be positively correlated with various indicators of negative outcome in most studies and this might also be true for the duration of untreated illness including the untreated prodromal phase.[6]

Thus by early detection – and treatment – of psychoses it is hoped to reduce the psychological, social and possibly biological disruption[7] that can lead to poor outcome.

Early detection of psychosis

Nowadays internationally employed definitions of the initial prodrome of psychosis or the 'at-risk mental state' are mainly based on attenuated psychotic symptoms (APS), brief limited intermittent psychotic symptoms (BLIPS) and a combination of trait and state risk factors, as developed at the Personal Assessment and Crisis Evaluation (PACE) clinic in Melbourne, Australia,[8] although their operationalization differs between centres (Table 10.1): whereas the Melbourne group[8] use the Brief Psychiatric Rating Scale (BPRS)[9] the Early Detection and Intervention Evaluation (EDIE) Trial group from Manchester, UK,[10] work with the Positive And Negative Syndrome Scale (PANSS)[11] and the Prevention through Risk Identification, Management and Education (PRIME) group from New Haven, USA, have developed a special instrument, the Structured Interview for/Scale Of Prodromal Syndromes (SIPS/SOPS).[12]

Despite applying the same criteria at first sight, i.e. APS, BLIPS and trait-state risk factors, the 12-month transition rates reported by these three groups differ. Figure 10.2 shows the transition data from the PACE prediction study of patients who had met criteria of an at-risk mental state and were only monitored for their symptoms,[8] from a recent intervention study by the same group that compared special pharmacological and psychological intervention to non-specific need-based intervention and, furthermore, distinguished between patients with full, partial and no compliance with medication,[14] from the EDIE trial studying cognitive therapy versus therapy as usual[10] and from the PRIME validation study, in which no special treatment was applied and people were just followed up.[15] Most of the patients in all studies are reported to have been included on the basis of APS. Summarizing these data and taking into account all data with a 12-month follow-up, on average 27.0% of patients transited to a full-blown psychosis during this time. Excluding those who had received a special treatment, 36.7% transited to psychosis within 12 months, an even higher number.

Thus, by employing transient or attenuated psychotic symptoms or the trait-state criterion, i.e. the Melbourne criteria, an early detection, and treatment, of psychosis prior to the first acute episode seem to target the late prodromal course when psychosis is imminent and social deficits are likely to have occurred already (Figure 10.3). Furthermore, it is arguable whether frank but transient psychotic symptoms, which would meet DSM-IV criteria of psychotic disorder Not Otherwise Specified (NOS) (298.9), really offer the opportunity for an intervention in psychosis that can truly be called early and preventive. In consequence, to detect psychosis that is earlier in the prodromal phase and, probably, before the onset or at least at the early stage of functional deficits, different criteria are needed.

In our prospective Cologne Early Recognition (CER) study, self-experienced, very early and subclinical symptoms, so called basic symptoms, according to the Bonn Scale for the Assessment of Basic Symptoms (BSABS)[16] were examined for their schizophrenia-predictive value.[17] About half of the

Table 10.1 Operationalizations of early detection and intervention study intake criteria

	PACE Phillips et al. (2000)[8]	*EDIE* Morrison et al. (2002)[10]	*PRIME* McGlashan et al. (2003)[13]
Attenuated psychotic symptoms (APS)	Magical thinking, ideas of reference (BPRS: unusual thought content – UTC score 2–3) Paranoid ideation (BPRS: suspiciousness score 3) Perceptual disturbances (BPRS: hallucination score 1–2) Odd thinking and speech (BPRS: conceptual disorganization score 1–3)	Delusions (PANSS: P1, P5 score 3) Suspiciousness (PANSS: P6 score 3–4) Hallucinations (PANSS: P3 score 2–3) Conceptual disorganization (PANSS: P2 score 3–4)	Unusual thought content/delusional ideas (SOPS: P1 score 3–5) Grandiosity (SOPS: P3 score 3–5) Suspiciousness/persecutory ideas (SOPS: P2 score 3–5) Perceptual abnormalities/hallucinations (SOPS: P4 score 3–5) Disorganized communication (SOPS: P5 score 3–5)
General requirements for APS	UTC held with a reasonable degree of conviction, frequency of several times per week, present for at least 1 week within the past year and not more than 5 years	Occurrence with a frequency of several times per week and change in mental state present for 1 week	Development/increase in severity within the past year and average frequency of at least once per week in the past month
Brief limited intermittent psychotic symptoms (BLIPS)	Magical thinking, ideas of reference (BPRS: unusual thought content – UTC score ≥ 4)	Delusions (PANSS: P1, P5 score 4–7)	Unusual thought content/delusional ideas (SOPS: P1 score 6) Grandiosity (SOPS: P3 score 6)

	Paranoid ideation (BPRS: suspiciousness score ≥ 4) Perceptual disturbances (BPRS: hallucination score ≥ 3) Odd thinking and speech (BPRS: conceptual disorganization score ≥4)	Suspiciousness (PANSS: P6 score 5–7) Hallucinations (PANSS: P3 score 4–7)	Suspiciousness/persecutory ideas (SOPS: P2 score 6) Perceptual abnormalities/hallucinations (SOPS: P4 score 6) Disorganized communication (SOPS: P5 score 6)
General requirements for BLIPS	UTC held with strong conviction, duration of episode less than a week, symptoms spontaneously resolve, occurrence within the past year	Present for less than 1 week prior to spontaneous resolution	Development within the past 3 months, no less than several minutes a day, at least once per month and no more than 1 hour a day for 4 days a week (on average) for 1 month, symptoms not seriously disorganizing or dangerous
Trait-state risk factor	First-degree relative with a psychotic disorder or schizotypal personality disorder or patient has a schizotypal personality disorder and reduction of functioning on the GAF scale of at least 30 points from premorbid level for at least 1 month and not more than 5 years	Family history of psychosis or patient has a schizotypal personality disorder and functional deterioration	First-degree relative with any psychotic disorder or patient has a schizotypal personality disorder according to DSM-IV and reduction of functioning on the GAF scale of at least 30 points for at least 1 month as compared to 12 months ago

PACE, Personal Assessment and Crisis Evaluation; EDIE, Early Detection and Intervention Evaluation Trial; PRIME, Prevention through Risk Identification, and Management and Education; BPRS, Brief Psychiatric Rating Scale; PANSS, Positive and Negative Syndrome Scale; SOPS, Scale of Prodromal Syndromes; GAF, Global Assessment of Functioning

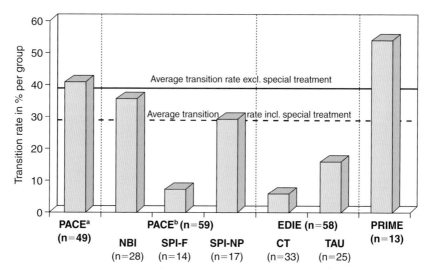

Figure 10.2 *12-month transition rates to psychosis employing the Melbourne criteria. PACE[a]: Prediction study,[8] monitoring PACE[b]: Intervention study,[14] NBI, unspecific need-based intervention; SPI, specific preventive pharmacological and psychotherapeutic intervention; F, fully compliant to medication; NP, non or only partially compliant to medication.*
EDIE: Intervention study,[10] CT, specific cognitive therapy; TAU, unspecific treatment as usual. PRIME: Validation study,[15] monitoring.

160 patients who were followed up (n = 79) – no patient had shown any psychotic symptoms at the first examination – developed schizophrenia during the average follow-up period of 9.6 years. Only two of those who transited to schizophrenia had not reported any basic symptom at first examination, but 33 of the 110 who did so did not develop schizophrenia. A transition to schizophrenia took place on average 1.9 ± 2.5 years after the first examination, the average duration of the prodrome from first reported basic symptom until first reported psychotic symptom was 5.6 ± 5.1 years. So as regards the presence of any basic symptom, the BSABS showed a high sensitivity (0.98), good specificity (0.59), good positive (0.70) and excellent negative predictive value (0.96), few false negative predictions (1.3%) but 20.6% false positive predictions. When looking at the prognostic accuracy of single basic symptoms at the time of the first interview, early self-experienced deficit of thought processing and perception were present among the later schizophrenics with a frequency that nearly satisfied the criterion of diagnostically relevant psychotic symptoms as proposed by Andreasen and Flaum (Table 10.2).[18] These 10 basic symptoms also showed quite a high positive predictive value along with high specificity, low

Table 10.2 Prognostic accuracy measures of basic symptoms with good positive predictive power and an occurrence in at least a quarter of patients later developing schizophrenia[17]

Basic symptom	Sensitivity	Specificity	PPV	NPV	PDLR	NDLR	OR	% FP	% FN
Thought interference	0.42	0.91	0.83	0.62	4.67	0.64	7.32	4.4	28.8
Thought perseveration	0.32	0.88	0.71	0.57	2.67	0.77	3.45	6.3	33.8
Thought pressure	0.38	0.96	0.91	0.62	9.50	0.65	14.71	1.9	30.6
Thought blockages	0.34	0.86	0.71	0.57	2.43	0.77	3.16	6.9	32.5
Disturbance of receptive language	0.39	0.91	0.82	0.61	4.33	0.67	6.46	4.4	30.0
Decreased ability to discriminate between ideas and perception, fantasy and true memories	0.27	0.95	0.84	0.57	5.40	0.77	7.03	2.5	36.3
Unstable ideas of reference	0.39	0.89	0.78	0.60	3.55	0.69	5.17	5.6	30.0
Derealization	0.28	0.90	0.73	0.56	2.80	0.80	3.50	5.0	35.6
Visual perception disturbances[a]	0.46	0.85	0.75	0.62	3.07	0.64	4.83	7.5	26.9
Acoustic perception disturbances[a]	0.29	0.89	0.72	0.53	2.64	0.80	3.30	5.6	35.0

[a] Rated as binary variable: 'at least any one present' versus 'none present'.

PPV, positive predictive value; NPV, negative predictive value; PDLR, positive diagnostic likelihood ratio; NDLR, negative diagnostic likelihood ratio; OR, odds ratio; %FP, % false positive predictions; %FN, % false negative predictions.

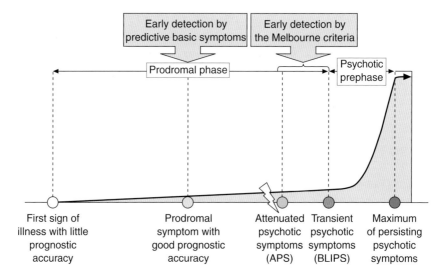

Figure 10.3 *Symptom development in psychosis: time-related model of the onset of symptom groups and starting points for early detection – and intervention.*

number of false positive predictions and positive likelihood ratio at least indicating small but probably important changes in pre-test probability (Table 10.2).[19] Thus, the accuracy of the prediction of schizophrenia – and not only of any psychotic disorder – by basic symptoms is easily comparable with that reported for positive symptoms for schizophrenia. Therefore, these 10 basic symptoms seem to offer a reasonable starting point for earlier detection; this is supported by the ABC study, in which 'trouble with thinking and concentration' including these cognitive basic symptoms occurs quite early and often at the very beginning of the prodromal phase.[1]

Adding these 10 basic symptoms to Figure 10.3, it seems possible to shift early detection and treatment of psychosis to a much earlier point and maybe even before the onset of social deficits.

Conclusion

To conclude, prediction of psychosis is not only necessary but also possible because:

- results of current studies with attenuated and transient psychotic symptoms indicate quite a high transition rate to psychosis of 36.7% on average over 1 year when no special treatment is applied (Figure 10.2);

- results of the Cologne Early Recognition (CER) study show prognostic accuracies for a subgroup of self-experienced cognitive–perceptive disturbances that are comparable with the diagnostic accuracies reported for positive psychotic symptoms;[17] and
- persons who suffer from these symptoms seek help for it,[3,4] thus providing the opportunity to see them early.

However, further enhancement in the accuracy of the prediction of psychosis should be sought. Not only single symptoms should be studied, but also symptom and risk factor patterns. With an average duration of the prodrome of 5 years, persons at risk will have to be followed up for many years to avoid a premature assessment of false positives.

References

1. Häfner H, Maurer K, Löffler W, an der Heiden W, Könnecke R, Hambrecht M, The early course of schizophrenia. In: Häfner H (ed), *Risk and Protective Factors in Schizophrenia – Towards a Conceptual Model of the Disease Process*. Steinkopff, Darmstadt: 2002.
2. WHO (1988) World Health Organization. Psychiatric Disability Assessment Schedule (WHO/DAS). WHO, Geneva.
3. Addington J, van Mastrigt S, Hutchinson J, Addington D, Pathways to care: help seeking behaviour in first episode psychosis. *Acta Psychiatr Scand* 2002; **106**:358–364.
4. Phillips LJ, Yung AR, Hearn N, McFarlane C, Hallgreen M, McGorry PD, Preventive mental health care: accessing the target population. *Aust NZ J Psychiatr* 1999; **33**:912–917.
5. Häfner H, an der Heiden W, The course of schizophrenia in the light of modern follow-up studies: the ABC and WHO studies. *Eur Arch Psychiatry Clin Neurosci* 1999; **249(Suppl 4)**:IV/14–IV/26.
6. Norman RMG, Malla AK, Duration of untreated psychosis: a critical examination of the concept and its importance. *Psychol Med* 2001; **31**:381–400.
7. Pantelis C, Velakoulis D, McGorry PD et al, Neuroanatomical abnormalities before and after onset of psychosis: a cross-sectional and longitudinal MRI comparison. *Lancet* 2003; **361**:281–288.
8. Phillips LJ, Yung AR, McGorry PD, Identification of young people at risk of psychosis: validation of Personal Assessment and Crisis Evaluation Clinic intake criteria. *Aust NZ J Psychiatry* 2000; **34(Suppl)**:S164–S169.
9. Overall JE, Gorham DR, The Brief Psychiatric Rating Scale. *Psychol Rep* 1962; **10**:799–812.
10. Morrison T, Bentall R, French P, Kilcommons A, Green J, Lewis S, Early detection and intervention for psychosis in primary care. *Acta Psychiatr Scand* 2002; **413**:44.
11. Kay SR, Fiszbein A, Opler LA, The Positive and Negative Syndrome Scale (PANSS) for schizophrenia. *Schizophr Bull* 1987; **13**:261–276.
12. Miller TJ, McGlashan TH, Woods SW et al, Symptom assessment in schizophrenic prodromal states. *Psychiatr Quarterly* 1999; **70**:273–287.
13. McGlashan TH, Zipursky RB, Perkins D et al, The Prime North America

randomized double-blind clinical trial of olanzapine versus placebo in patients at risk of being prodromally symptomatic for psychosis. I. Study rationale and design. *Schizophr Res* 2003; **61**:7–18.

14. McGorry PD, Yung AR, Phillips LJ et al, A randomized controlled trial of interventions designed to reduce the risk of progression to first-episode psychosis in a clinical sample with subthreshold symptoms. *Arch Gen Psychiatry* 2002; **59**:921–928.

15. Miller TJ, McGlashan TH, Lifshey Rosen J et al, Prospective diagnosis of the initial prodrome for schizophrenia based on the Structured Interview for Prodromal Syndromes: preliminary evidence of interrater reliability and predictive validity. *Am J Psychiatry* 2002; **159**:863–865.

16. Gross G, Huber G, Klosterkötter J, Linz M, *Bonner Skala für die Beurteilung von Basissymptomen* (BSABS; Bonn Scale for the Assessment of Basic Symptoms). Springer: Berlin Heidelberg New York, 1987.

17. Klosterkötter J, Hellmich M, Steinmeyer EM, Schultze-Lutter F, Diagnosing schizophrenia in the initial prodromal phase. *Arch Gen Psychiatry* 2001; **58**:158–164.

18. Andreasen NC, Flaum M, Schizophrenia. The characteristic symptoms. *Schizophr Bull* 1991; **17**:27–49.

19. Jaeschko R, Guyatt GH, Sackett DL, User's guides to the medical literature. III. How to use an article about a diagnostic test. B. What are the results and will they help me in caring for my patients? *JAMA* 1994; **271**:703–707.

chapter 11

The use of concepts in relation to early intervention in psychosis: a critical discussion

Tor K Larsen

The idea of early intervention in psychosis has emerged and developed rapidly during the past decade – a kind of 'movement' seemed to develop with the energetic Professor Patrick McGorry from Melbourne, Australia, as its initiator. Meetings of the International Early Psychosis Association (IEPA) are arranged regularly and early-detection services are evolving all over the world. The idea of early intervention has brought new concepts into the field of psychiatric discourse on psychosis, such as primary prevention, at-risk mental states, etc. This calls for analysis of the concepts that are being used. This chapter is largely based on a review on conceptual and ethical problems related to early intervention and/or prevention of psychosis by Heinemaa and Larsen,[1] published recently in *Current Opinion in Psychiatry*. Some aspects will be elaborated and a new concept (hypopsychosis) related to the description of possible presages to psychosis will be introduced.

The discussion will focus on basic concepts that we use and develop when we talk about early intervention in psychosis and some key concepts will be discussed in more depth. These concepts are the brief limited intermittent psychotic states (BLIPS) and the idea of false positives. Early psychosis is often divided into phases such as the prodromal phase, the duration of untreated psychosis (DUP) and treated psychosis (Figure 11.1).

When talking about early detection, one could either focus on the reduction of DUP (secondary prevention), or try to intervene before the

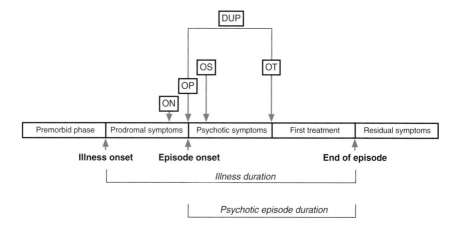

Figure 11.1 *Early course of psychosis. (Modified from Larsen TK et al. Schizophr Bull 1996; 22:241–256.[2]) ON, onset of negative symptoms; OP, onset of psychosis, positive symptoms; OS, onset of psychotic syndrome; OT, onset of treatment; DUP, duration of untreated psychosis.*

onset of psychosis at the so-called prodromal stage (primary prevention). In the early Treatment and Intervention in Psychosis Study (TIPS) a reduction in DUP from 26 weeks (median) before any early-detection strategies were developed (historical control sample 1993–94), to 4, 5 weeks (median) was achieved with the use of early-detection strategies (early-detection sample), such as education campaigns and low-threshold detection teams.[3] Receiving early treatment was significantly correlated with fewer symptoms and better social functioning at the start of treatment and currently a 1, 2, 5 and 10 year follow-up of the sample is being carried out to study whether early detection has a lasting effect on outcome.

In Stavanger, Norway, (the early-intervention site of TIPS) a clinic has been established for those that have psychosis-like symptoms, but do not fulfil the criteria for full-blown psychosis according to the TIPS inclusion criteria (which is equivalent to 'psychosis' according to DSM-IV, see discussion later). At this early Treatment Of PrePsychosis (TOPP) clinic, we treat individuals without antipsychotic medications and it has been experienced that intensive psychotherapy might prevent development of psychosis. In the first 14 cases detected during the first 2 years we found a transition rate to psychosis of about 40% within the first year. In the past 2 years two skilled psychologists have been employed, who are treating these cases very intensively with psychotherapy and out of the last 10 cases followed for 1 year, only one showed transition to psychosis. These data are of course preliminary, on small samples and must be interpreted with caution, but raise the question of whether medication is the only way to prevent psychosis from developing.

When working with these possibly prepsychotic people a significant problem is encountered related to which concepts one should use. Concepts that imply, with absolute necessity, an upcoming transition to psychosis are problematic because if the preventive strategies work, the patients will not develop what is prevented. Being stigmatized as possibly (probably?) prepsychotic might be harmful for some patients. It must be taken into consideration that people who fulfil criteria for prepsychosis must be expected to have a higher rate of close relatives with severe mental disorders and, despite recent anti-stigma campaigns, the popular myths about psychosis and schizophrenia are still very pessimistic.[4] Examples of such invalid concepts are 'prepsychosis, pre-schizophrenia and prodromal symptoms'. Many studies and manuals are, however, still using these concepts and it seems difficult to discover better concepts and avoid misunderstandings. All these concepts are truly retrospective and should be avoided. How then should one label the people who are included in studies of primary prevention of psychosis? In order to come up with better alternatives we need to take a close look at what clinical syndromes the different tentative presages to psychosis consist of, i.e. are we treating people who have developed some kind of symptoms or are they non-symptomatic high risk cases?

The concept 'at-risk mental state' was developed by the Melbourne group; this is a key concept in the Comprehensive Assessment of At Risk Mental States (CAARMS)[5] and forms a conceptual basis for a number of other instruments describing prepsychosis. The problem with this term is that it should really be called 'at-risk of psychosis mental state'. If the word 'psychosis' is not included, it is unclear what kind of risk is involved. The most frequently used scale for describing prepsychotic stages is probably the Structured Interview for Prodromal Syndromes (SIPS) developed by the PRIME group.[6] SIPS incorporates many of the ideas developed by the thorough studies in Germany[7] and the Bonn Scale of Basic Symptoms (BSABS). SIPS defines three prodromal states that correspond well to the syndromes in the CAARMS and definitions are given in Box 11.1.

Box 11.1 Structured Interview for Prodromal Syndromes (SIPS) criteria for prodromal syndromes

(A) Brief intermittent psychotic syndrome

Positive symptoms at psychotic intensity are present, but they are not disorganizing or dangerous or do not last for at least 1 hour per day at an average frequency of 4 days per week over 1 month. If the psychotic intensity symptoms have never been present at that frequency, but have begun in the past 3 months and are currently present at least several minutes a day at a frequency of at least once per month, the criteria for this prodromal syndrome are met

(B) Attenuated positive prodromal syndrome

The prodromal or attenuated positive symptoms are found on scales P1–P5 of the Scale of prodromal symptoms (SOPS). A score of 3, 4, or 5 on any symptom scale defines the prodromal level of intensity. If any of the symptoms have begun in the past year or currently rate at least one scale point higher compared to 12 months ago and occur at this level at an average frequency of at least once per week in the past month, the criteria for this prodromal syndrome are met

(C) Genetic risk and deterioration syndrome

Consists of a combined genetic risk for a schizophrenic spectrum disorder and recent functional deterioration. The genetic risk criteria can be met if the patient has a first-degree relative with any psychotic disorder (affective or non-affective) and/or the patient meets DSM-IV schizotypal personality disorder criteria. Functional deterioration is operationally defined as a 30% or greater drop in the Global Assessment of Functioning (GAF) score during the past month compared with 12 months ago

A critique of the concept 'brief intermittent psychotic state'

Recent studies on primary prevention of psychosis have clearly found that few patients with the genetic high risk and recent psychosocial deterioration subtypes are detected, they simply do not seem to be treatment seeking. In my view, the group of brief intermittent psychotic states should not to be included at all as a possible prodromal state. Both McGlashan and McGorry state that the brief psychosis subtype 'do not meet the DSM-IV duration criteria for psychosis', but the most unspecific concept of psychosis in DSM-IV – the psychosis Not Otherwise Specified (NOS) – does not give any duration criteria whatsoever. The criteria read: 'This category includes psychotic symptomatology (i.e. delusions, hallucinations, disorganized speech, grossly disorganized or catatonic behaviour) about which there is inadequate information to make a specific diagnosis or about which there is contradictory information, or disorders with psychotic symptoms that do not meet the criteria for any specific psychotic disorder'.[8] The way we understand these criteria, any psychotic condition even with extremely short duration, should fall in this category. Psychosis NOS thus comprises both early-detected psychosis and possible 'benign' forms of psychosis that probably do not need any treatment at all. Under any circumstances it would be conceptually wrong to classify them as prodromal or prepsychotic. The consequence of this critique ought to be conceived at a conceptual and not necessarily at a clinical level. BLIPS should be understood as a psychotic condition, maybe in some instances as a benign subtype. BLIPS might be a presage to more severe (long-lasting) psychosis, but it is under no circumstances a pre- or hypopsychotic state and should be excluded from studies on primary prevention of psychosis.

A new concept – hypopsychosis

Since we regard the BLIPS as a per definition psychotic state and the genetic high risk group seems to be very rare in studies of primary prevention of psychosis, we are left with only one group of possible prepsychotics from the SIPS-scale; the attenuated positive symptom state. This concept is too long to function as a diagnosis, it is more a description of the underlying psychopathology, but it also seems to imply that the symptoms have been more severe earlier on, which is very often not the case. A more brief concept and one that is more adequately related to the clinical picture that we see in these cases is needed. I believe that a better concept for this condition is *hypopsychosis* because it emphasizes the fact that these patients are treatment seeking and ill, and that we are dealing with a clinical condition, much like we understand hypomania as related to mania. Hypopsychosis might develop into manifest psychosis or it might vanish in time or as a consequence of some sort of treatment. In our clinic hypopsychosis is treated with supportive psychotherapy and rehabilitation, but in other studies antipsychotic medication might emerge as effective. Even a concept such as 'antipsychotics' is a construct developed to label medication that is effective in the treatment of psychosis. If research shows that antipsychotics are effective also for hypopsychosis it may be better to label these drugs *neuromodulators*, taking this effect into consideration. Ongoing studies with sound scientific designs (randomized and double blind) will reveal more about the effect of neuromodulators such as antipsychotics on hypopsychosis; only with time will we be able to judge what the best treatment will be. One advantage with the concept of hypopsychosis is that it can be understood as a condition that might need treatment in itself – it is not a condition that necessarily will develop into something more severe. Patients who are treated for hypopsychosis can conceptualize and understand the treatment given with the specific aim of reducing the symptoms that were present and not only in order to prevent something in the future. Even patients who never develop a more serious condition can receive treatment within this paradigm.

The problem with 'false positives'

Another concept that is often used in a confusing manner in discussions on prevention of psychosis is the 'false positives'. False positives are used to characterize those cases that fulfil criteria for some tentative prepsychotic condition, but never develop (or would have developed) psychosis. Normally false positiveness means cases in which a screening test gives a false suspicion of the underlying disorder we are screening for. An example would be a blood test for some infection, but when we carry out more thorough tests, we have a negative result. Whether a condition (hypopsychosis) develops into another disorder (psychosis) has nothing to do with false positives, but rather to which degree the first condition is a presage to the second (predictive power). False positive cases of hypopsychosis would be cases in which a positive screening test for hypopsychosis proved to be false when we carried out a more complete assessment.

Concluding remarks

In general the field of research regarding primary prevention of psychosis seems to be making significant progress. There are several ongoing and promising studies from which we expect to learn more about whether it really is possible to detect and treat people who are at the edge of developing psychosis. The most promising studies are being carried out in Australia (the PACE clinic, McGorry's group) and in the USA (the PRIME clinic, McGlashan's group), but sound studies are also being carried out in the UK, in the Netherlands, Germany and in Scandinavian countries. It is, however, very important that there is a thorough discussion of both ethical and conceptual problems related to primary prevention of psychosis in order to avoid the establishment of treatment and detection initiatives that are not ethically or clinically sound. The labelling of non-psychotic people as 'possibly psychotic', 'prepsychotic', 'preschizophrenic' or 'at risk of developing psychosis' is controversial. It should be borne in mind that the diagnosis should be for the benefit of the people. We believe that the introduction of the concept 'hypopsychosis' can bring the field forward somewhat; hypopsychosis is a clinical condition (defined in manuals such as SIPS) that needs treatment, which often (probably in almost 50% of the cases) can be a presage to psychosis. The concept does not label people as having early psychosis, but a weak form of psychosis. Hypopsychosis is much similar to hypomania, a concept that has not created much clinical or conceptual controversy. Perhaps hypopsychosis is a rather benign condition that does not always require therapy. People with hypopsychosis who are included in studies on primary prevention should be both treatment seeking and worried that their problems might develop into something more severe and disabling. We argue that BLIPS should be understood and treated as a psychotic condition and not as prepsychosis, and there should be a more unambiguous use of other key concepts such as false positives and primary prevention in general. Finally, we believe that ongoing research soon will be able to develop a more valid description of hypopsychosis and we support any attempt that aims to bring more clarity to this promising field of clinical research.

References

1. Heinemaa M, Larsen TK, Psychosis: conceptual and ethical aspects of early diagnosis and intervention. *Curr Opin Psychiatry* 2002; **15**:533–541.
2. Larsen TK, McGlashan TH, Moe LC, First episode schizophrenia. I Early course parameters. *Schizophr Bull* 1996; **22**:241–256.
3. Larsen TK, McGlashan TH, Johannessen JO et al, Shortened duration of untreated first episode of psychosis: changes in patient characteristics at treatment. *Am J Psychiatry* 2001; **158**:1917–1919.
4. Larsen TK, Opjordsmoen S, Early identification and treatment of schizophrenia: conceptual and ethical considerations. *Psychiatry* 1996; **59**:371–380.
5. McGorry PD, Preventive strategies in early psychosis: verging on reality. *Br J Psychiatry Suppl* 1998; **172**:1–2.
6. Miller TJ, McGlashan TH, Rosen JL et al, Prospective diagnosis of the initial prodrome for schizophrenia based on the Structured Interview for Prodromal

Syndromes: preliminary evidence of interrater reliability and predictive validity. *Am J Psychiatry* 2002; **159**:863–865.

7. Huber G, Gross G, The concept of basic symptoms in schizophrenic and schizo-affective psychoses. *Recenti Prog Med* 1989; **80**:646–652.

8. American Psychiatric Association. DSM-IV, *Diagnostic and Statistical Manual of Mental Disorders*. (4th edn). American Psychiatric Association: Washington, DC, 1994.

chapter 12

Is the relationship between duration of untreated psychosis and outcome a result of premorbid deficits?

Hélène Verdoux and Audrey Cougnard

A cornerstone argument supporting early detection is drawn from studies that have investigated the links between duration of untreated psychosis (DUP) and prognosis and reported that subjects with a long DUP have a poorer clinical outcome than those with a shorter delay between onset of psychosis and first treatment.[1,2] The rationale for early intervention is that reducing DUP may have a favourable impact on the subsequent course of the illness. However, the existence of a causal link between DUP and outcome is not perfectly estab-lished, as these findings are from observational studies where the delay between onset of psychosis and first treatment was not randomly distributed with regard to the other characteristics of the disease. Thus, factors delaying treatment seeking, such as poor premorbid adjustment or severe negative symptoms, may also independently predict poor outcome. Hence, the association between DUP and poor outcome may be a spurious one, confounded by these factors.[2–5]

Characteristics associated with duration of untreated psychosis

The first question is to assess what characteristics are associated with DUP in naturalistic settings. This issue was explored by us in the Bordeaux First

Episode study.[6] This population-based study was carried out on first-admitted subjects presenting with psychotic symptoms consecutively hospitalized in the acute wards of Bordeaux's psychiatric hospital serving an urban geographical area with 250 000 inhabitants. DUP was categorized according to the median into 'short' DUP (< 3 months) versus 'long' (≥ 3 months) DUP. Univariate analyses showed that patients with a long DUP were more likely to have a low educational level, to have had poorer global functioning in the previous year, and to present with a more severe global clinical state and more prominent negative symptoms at admission. A long delay was also associated with a diagnosis of schizophrenia broadly defined, and with a family history of psychiatric hospitalization in first and/or second-degree relatives. Multivariate analyses were then used to explore which characteristics independently predicted a long delay between onset of first psychotic symptoms and first treatment. Four such characteristics were found independently: family history of psychiatric hospitalization (adjusted odds ratio (OR) = 12.1, 95% confidence interval (CI) 1.15 to 97.0, $P = 0.02$), a low educational level (adjusted OR = 7.7, 95% CI 1.0 to 50.0, $P = 0.05$), a low Global Assessment of Functioning Score during the previous year (adjusted OR = 0.93, 95% CI 0.86 to 0.99, $P = 0.04$) and, at trend level, a high Clinical Global Impression score (measuring severity of illness) at admission (adjusted OR = 4.0, 95% CI 0.87 to 18.3, $P = 0.07$). No interaction was found between these variables. Thus subjects with a long DUP are already different from the other subjects when presenting for treatment for the first time, and importantly, the characteristics differentiating those subjects have also been found to be associated with poor outcome in previous studies.

To explore whether or not the association between DUP and outcome was confounded by these characteristics the subjects were followed up over a 2-year period.[7] In accordance with most other studies it was found that subjects with a long DUP were much more likely to have a chronic course of illness, that is no remission of psychotic symptoms over the 2-year follow-up. An assessment was done of whether the strength of the association between duration of psychosis before admission and chronic course of psychosis over the follow-up was modified after adjustment for potential confounders measured at first admission. The strength of the association between DUP and chronic course of psychosis over the follow-up was strongly reduced (by 63%) after adjustment for premorbid functioning in the year preceding admission. The effect sizes of the association were also reduced after adjustment for the severity of illness at first admission and for

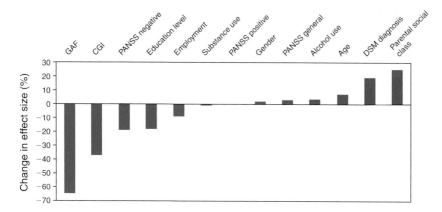

Figure 12.1 *Change in the effect size (%) of the association between DUP and chronicity of psychosis after adjustment for explanatory factors. GAF, Global Assessment of Functioning; CGI, Clinical Global Impression scale; PANSS, Positive And Negative Syndrome Scale; DSM diagnosis: schizophrenia broadly defined vs other. (From Verdoux H et al.* Schizophr Res 2001; **49**:231–241.[7]

the intensity of negative symptoms. There was no major change in the effect sizes after adjustment for positive symptoms, educational level and employment status (Figure 12.1).

Association between duration of untreated psychosis and outcome

What is the most likely explanation for the findings discussed above? The first explanation is that the association between DUP and poor outcome is a spurious one, confounded by the fact that poor premorbid functioning (severity of illness/intensity of negative symptoms) is independently associated with both DUP and poor outcome, with no direct causal link between these two latter variables. If this hypothesis were true, reducing DUP would have no impact on the subsequent course of the illness. The second hypothesis is that DUP is on the causal pathway between poor premorbid functioning and poor outcome. Subjects with poor premorbid functioning may be less likely to seek treatment when they become ill, and because of this delayed treatment they are subsequently at increased risk of presenting with a chronic course of illness. In other words, DUP may at least in part mediate the association between poor premorbid adjustment and poor prognosis. If this hypothesis is true, shortening DUP may contribute to reducing the risk of no remission of psychotic symptoms. At this time it is still not possible to conclude on the basis of available findings whether the association between DUP and outcome is a causal one, or may be better explained by the fact that the factors delaying treatment seeking are also independently predicting poor outcome.

The impact of DUP on the natural course of psychosis, mediated by a putative neurotoxicity of untreated psychosis,[1] is as yet a speculative hypothesis. To date, there is only one study by the Australian group[9] showing that subjects with a long DUP have poorer cognitive functioning. To our knowledge, no other study investigating that issue has reported an association between long DUP and poorer cognitive function or more brain structural abnormalities. There is more convincing evidence regarding the short-term benefits of early treatment, by reducing at-risk behaviour such as self-harm, aggressiveness, substance use, disruption of social network and educational trajectory.[8,10-13] However, although early treatment may have obvious short-term benefits at an individual level, it is far from established that reducing DUP is more beneficial than risky in a public health perspective, i.e. at the level of the community.[14-16]

References

1. Lieberman J, Perkins D, Belger A et al, The early stages of schizophrenia: speculations on pathogenesis, pathophysiology, and therapeutic approaches. *Biol Psychiatry* 1999; **50**:884–897.
2. Norman R, Malla AK, Duration of untreated psychosis: a critical examination of the concept and its importance. *Psychol Med* 2001; **31**:381–400.
3. Larsen TK, McGlashan TH, Johannessen JO et al, Shortened duration of untreated first episode of psychosis: changes in patient characteristics at treatment. *Am J Psychiatry* 2001; **158**:1917–1919.
4. McGlashan TH, Duration of untreated psychosis in first-episode schizophrenia: marker or determinant of course? *Biol Psychiatry* 1999; **46**:899–907.
5. Warner R, The prevention of schizophrenia: what interventions are safe and effective? *Schizophr Bull* 2001; **27**:551–562.
6. Verdoux H, Bergey C, Assens F et al, Prediction of duration of psychosis before first admission. *Eur Psychiatry* 1998; **13**:346–352.
7. Verdoux H, Liraud F, Bergey C, Assens F, Abalan F, van Os J, Is the association between duration of untreated psychosis and outcome confounded? A two-year follow-up study of first-admitted patients. *Schizophr Res* 2001; **49**:231–241.
8. Verdoux H, Liraud F, Gonzales B, Assens F, Abalan F, van Os J, Predictors and outcome characteristics associated with suicidal behaviour in early psychosis: a two-year follow-up of first-admitted subjects. *Acta Psychiatr Scand* 2001; **103**:347–354.
9. Amminger G, Edwards J, Brewer W, Harrigan S, McGorry P, Duration of untreated psychosis and cognitive deterioration in first-episode schizophrenia. *Schizophr Res* 2002; **54**:223–230.

10. Courtenay K, First episode psychosis. GPs must assess patients' risk behaviour. *BMJ* 2002; **324**:976.
11. McGlashan TH, Miller TJ, Woods SW, Pre-onset detection and intervention research in schizophrenia psychoses: current estimates of benefit and risk. *Schizophr Bull* 2001; **27**:563–570.
12. Sandor A, Courtenay K, First episode psychosis. Patients must be asked about suicidal ideation and substance misuse. *BMJ* **324**:976.
13. Verdoux H, Liraud F, Gonzales B, Assens F, Abalan F, van Os J, Suicidality and substance misuse in first-admitted subjects with psychotic disorder. *Acta Psychiatr Scand* 1999; **100**:389–395.
14. Cougnard A, Salmi R, Verdoux H, A decade of debate on early intervention in psychosis: a systematic review of criteria for assessing screening usefulness. *Schizophr Res* 2003; **60**:91–93.
15. Verdoux H, Have the times come for early intervention in psychosis? *Acta Psychiatr Scand* 2001; **103**:321–322.
16. Verdoux H, Cougnard A, The early detection and treatment controversy in schizophrenia research. *Curr Opin Psychiatry* 2003; **16**:175–179.

chapter 13

Is early intervention a waste of valuable resources?

Anthony S David

The current status of early intervention is reflected in the following quotations.

> The first meeting [of the European First Episode Schizophrenia Network, in 1995] . . . was hosted by Robin Murray's department in London and was attended by 20 people from 4 European countries. Its most recent meeting in Switzerland [Feb 2002] was attended by over 100 delegates from 16 countries
>
> Shôn Lewis, *British Journal of Psychiatry (Suppl)*, 2002[1]

> Potential benefits of prepsychotic intervention: patients more easily engaged . . . develop trust . . . minimal DUP, reduced comorbidity . . . inpatient care; psychosocial impact minimized; . . . delay or avoid 1st psychotic episode. May prove highly cost-effective . . .
>
> McGorry et al, *Archives of General Psychiatry*, 2002[2]

It is now government policy in England to have a psychosis early-intervention service. The blueprint for the National Health Service (NHS) called the NHS Plan[3] says about early intervention: 'it reduces the period of untreated psychosis', and therefore '50 early intervention teams will be established' and that, 'by 2004, all young people who experience their first episode of psychosis will receive the early intensive support they need', and £50 million of new money is being put towards it.

The idea of early intervention seems to come from general medicine. There are medical truisms, such as:

- Prevention is better than cure.

- 'A stitch in time saves nine'
- The earlier we start treatment, the less the illness will progress.

Requirements of effective early intervention

The above 'theoretical' arguments are uncontroversial. Putting theory into practice requires a few extra steps (see Chapter 12). In order to make early intervention effective, there are a number of prerequisites, which could be taken from any textbook of social medicine or epidemiology and could be applied to any medical condition. The following conditions are necessary for early intervention to be useful:

- a population-based strategy
- easy identification of cases in the population
- highly specific and sensitive case finding
- interventions which are relatively non-invasive with minimal side effects
- demonstrably clear benefits of early treatment
- cost effectiveness.

That is the challenge that early intervention schemes set themselves.

For the sake of argument suppose all the studies that are in progress have now been completed and the data published and put together in a systematic review. There are about seven large trials throughout the UK with very large numbers – half a million participants in total (longstanding, long duration, longitudinal studies). The results show the odds ratio is 1.01 with 95% confidence interval (CI) 0.99 to 1.03. As can be seen, the confidence intervals include possible worthwhile effects as well as possible detrimental effects. It seems that even with the large number of participants, the trials are underpowered. In fact, these figures are real but they have nothing to do with psychosis. They are figures for screening for breast cancer with mammography published in 2001 by the Cochrane Collaboration,[4] which were of course controversial. However, this is the paradigm case for early intervention in medicine: early detection of breast cancer with mammography. But the odds ratio is 1.01. When considering schizophrenia versus cancer, it is clear that in the case of schizophrenia, there are severe difficulties with early identification of cases, high false positives and low false negatives, questionably effective treatment with minimal side effects, and unknown benefits of early treatment and cost effectiveness (see for example Woods et al[5]). Early intervention for psychosis is a new area, it is not something like breast cancer which is diagnosed under the microscope and can be removed with the surgeon's knife; diagnosing and treating schizophrenia early is much more complex.

Some data which illustrate the pitfalls of an early, broadly targeted intervention strategy are presented below. These come from a Swedish conscript survey, a population-based study, which examined genuinely pre-morbid social factors in 18-year-old men at the time of their conscription (Table 13.1).[6] The men who came out as most likely to develop schizophrenia up to approximately 15 years later were those who had fewer than two friends, preferring to socialize in small groups, were more sensitive than others and did not have a steady girlfriend. If all of those risk factors are present, for the chance of developing schizophrenia the odds ratio is 30. This is similar to having two parents with schizophrenia, it is more or less like having an identical twin with schizophrenia. So this is a powerful social risk factor and has been adjusted for family history. However, these factors together only account for very few cases of schizophrenia and are only present in 1% of the population. If one looks at just not having a girlfriend or not having any friends, separately, then we are talking about factors that are present in 20–40% of the population. So this is really a worthwhile target and it is accounting for many cases of schizophrenia. The odds ratios for individuals with two or more of these risk factors are still very high, and the amount of illness in the population thereby reduced if the number of friends people have was increased, would be quite substantial. And as far as I know there would be no side effects of such a treatment.

Attraction of early intervention services

Why is it then with all of the problems described above that clinicians seem to like early intervention? First, the patients are less ill, by definition, even if you take McGorry's group in Melbourne, Australia, who are at very high risk, the number needed to treat is 4 or more, according to his group's recent published study.[2] Thus four of the people one would treat would not normally develop psychosis. Even in the control group, only a third of the group are developing psychosis, so by definition, this is not an ill group. In my opinion, despite the fact that early intervention sounds like a rather good concept, in practice there are enough established cases of psychosis and these need our attention first. The various 'risky' mental states can be dealt with later.

Table 13.1 Swedish Conscript Cohort Study. Social and inter-personal variables and risk for schizophrenia

	No of variables[a]				
	0	*1*	*2*	*3*	*4*
No schizophrenia (n = 174)	10	49	58	42	15
% populations (n = 50 000)	21.0	44.1	26.9	7.0	1.0
Odds ratio (95% CI)	1.00	2.3 (1.1 to 4.9)	4.5 (2.2 to 9.4)	12.6 (6.1 to 26.7)	30.7 (12.9 to 73.8)
Population attributable fraction		16.1	25.9	22.2	8.3

Population attributable fraction is low despite greatly increased risk for schizophrenia of having 2 or more social risk factors (data from Malmberg et al[6]).
[a]Variables: <2 friends; preferring small groups; more sensitive than others; no steady girlfriend.

Those clinical teams who specialize in early intervention see patients who are, inevitably, younger, and find the work fulfilling. It is natural to feel more optimistic when dealing with younger people with psychosis. Early intervention services attract new resources, especially in the UK, so it is possible to recruit new staff who are optimistic and who want to work in this area. Such services are guaranteed research support and sponsorship. In generic services, all patients are ill by definition. Patients are old and they are getting older. Resources are diverted away from generic community teams to the new service in order to comply with the NHS Plan in England, and probably in other places in the world as well, so staff posts in generic services are hard to fill and staff burnout is high. It is very hard to get research support, to work on 'ordinary' patients with established illnesses and there is little chance of sponsorship from industry. Clinicians like early intervention services because they are able to 'pass on their failures'. After all of the experimental interventions have been done (with or without effect), and all the new monies are spent, and after all the reports have been written and published, when the patients are 35 years they are no longer of interest to early interventionists and the generic services have to take over.

There are some medical truisms we ignore at our peril:

- Continuity of care is paramount.
- Follow medical precedent (i.e., if it does not work in breast cancer, is it really going to work in schizophrenia?).
- First, do no harm.
- Triage, i.e. if a person is treatable, you treat the sickest first.

Problems with testing the early intervention hypothesis

There are at least two major problems with the objective testing of the hypothesis that 'early intervention in psychosis is effective'. The first is that the hypothesis is becoming irrefutable: if it is not working, it means enough has not been done, or, one did not intervene early enough. The second problem is that those carrying out the evaluation have an interest in its success.

In the quotations at the beginning of this chapter, Shon Lewis, in introducing a selection of commissioned articles, mentioned rightly that it was sponsored by a pharmaceutical company. McGorry quite rightly acknowledges the sponsorship of other drug companies in his publications. They are all very interested in this area, so early intervention is here to stay. Even if it is ineffective, it will not stop but may possibly lead to earlier and more elaborate interventions because it is government policy at present.

Early intervention is attractive to academics because publications and research funds are easily achieved. Clinicians find it appealing because it provides funds for them to improve their working conditions. Pharmaceutical companies like it because it has great potential to massively increase their markets and hence has their backing. Patients probably like it – although it is difficult to know for sure, as many patient organizations are now getting funding from the pharmaceutical industry. A lot of the work is based on patients who are help seeking, and they are a minority.

Alternatives to early intervention

Do we really need early intervention? Does it overemphasize the role of antipsychotic drugs? I would like to challenge the idea of 'corrosive pessimism' attributed to Kraepelin in the early 20th Century, to which early intervention services claim to be a response. Davis and colleagues did a meta-analysis of all the early studies of neuroleptic drugs; all drugs versus placebo in the treatment of schizophrenia.[7] They found that the likelihood that the effect was due to chance was less than 1 in 10 to the 36th power – or a billion billion billion billion. So where does the premise that schizophrenia is untreatable come from? And why has 'corrosive pessimism' taken hold? In fact, we have very good treatments. The analysis by Weiden and Olfson[8] suggests that if we make better use of the treatments we have, we can greatly improve the outcome of schizophrenia. Their analysis looked at relapse and drew upon the fact that people with schizophrenia discontinue their treatment early.

It is known that when patients discontinue treatment, 80% will relapse. Even under highly-controlled, well-managed conditions of a randomized controlled trial, continuous treatment is substantially better than intermittent treatment.[9] The relapse rates with continuous treatments are relatively low and they are three times greater in intermittent treatment, even when that is carried out under physician guidance, and even in first episode cases. Work from Robinson and colleagues[10] from the Hillside Hospital, Long Island, New York, is based on a middle-class population where they have an early intervention service. Even so, if patients are followed up after their first episode, by 5 years virtually all will have relapsed. And people who relapse tend to be those who do not take medication. In a recent European study[11] it was shown that relapse after a first episode is disappointingly high and is most strongly predicted by non-compliance.

Conclusions

From a dispassionate appraisal of the research literature on the treatment of schizophrenia, the most obvious and evidence-based target for interventions in schizophrenia is to prevent premature discontinuation of treatment and not early intervention. Efforts to help patients with established illness stay on their medication and in touch with services would have a dramatic impact on morbidity and we already have the evidence to prove this.[12,13] If an early intervention service is to be useful, it should be at the population level, free of side effects and inexpensive, and should not undermine clinical practice. On the basis of the Swedish data,[6] we might consider a befriending scheme.

As it stands there is only one possible conclusion: early intervention in schizophrenia is a waste of valuable resources.

References

1. Lewis S, The European first episode schizophrenia network. *Br J Psychiatr* 2002; **181**(Suppl 43):S1–S2.
2. McGorry PD, Yung AR, Phillips LJ et al, Randomized controlled trial of interventions designed to reduce the risk of progression to first-episode psychosis in a clinical sample with subthreshold symptoms. *Arch Gen Psychiatr* 2002; **59**:921–928.
3. Department of Health, *The NHS Plan*. Executive summary 2000. Crown Copyright.
4. Olsen O, Gotzsche PC, Screening for breast cancer with mammography. *Cochrane Database Syst Rev* 2001; (4):CD001877.
5. Woods SW, Miller TJ, Davidson L, Hawkins KA, Sernyak MJ, McGlashan TH, Estimated yield of early detection of prodromal or first episode patients by screening first degree relatives of schizophrenia patients. *Schizophr Res* 2001; **53**:21–27.
6. Malmberg A, Lewis G, David A, Allebeck P, Premorbid adjustment and personality in schizophrenia. *Br J Psychiatr* 1998; **172**:308–313.
7. Davis JM, Matalon L, Watanabe MD et al, Depot antipsychotic drugs. Place in therapy. *Drugs* 1994; **47**:741–773.
8. Weiden PJ, Olfson M, Cost of relapse in schizophrenia. *Schizophr Bull* 1995; **21**: 419–429.
9. Kane JM, Schizophrenia. *N Engl J Med* 1996; **334**:34–41
10. Robinson D, Woerner MG, Alvir JM et al, Predictors of relapse following response from a first episode of schizophrenia or schizoaffective disorder. *Arch Gen Psychiatr* 1999; **56**:241–247.

11. Novak-Grubic V, Tavcar R, Predictors of noncompliance in males with first-episode schizophrenia, schizophreniform and schizoaffective disorder. *Eur Psychiatry* 2002; **17**:148–154.
12. Kemp R, Kirov G, Everitt B et al, Randomised controlled trial of compliance therapy: 18 month follow-up. *Br J Psychiatr* 1998; **172**:413–419.
13. Kemp R, David AS, Patient compliance. In: Lieberman JA, Murray RM (eds), *Comprehensive Care of Schizophrenia*. Martin Dunitz: London, 2001.

chapter 14

Why antipsychotics are anti-'psychotic'

Shitij Kapur and David C Mamo

The history of the relation between dopamine, psychosis and antipsychotics starts with the discovery of antipsychotic drugs just over five decades ago. At that time psychological theories of schizophrenia were prominent, and major biological theories restricted to abnormal metabolism in the brain.[1,2] It was in this context that Delay et al reported the discovery of the antipsychotic actions of chlorpromazine,[3] followed by reports of the efficacy of reserpine in the treatment of a variety of serious psychiatric disorders.[4,5] However, these drugs were neither regarded as having specific efficacy in psychosis, nor restricted to the treatment of schizophrenia, assuming instead a broad indication as 'major tranquillizers'.[6]

Since then hundreds of compounds with putative antipsychotic activity have been synthesized and dozens have made it to the clinic, with the more novel agents called 'atypical' antipsychotics referring to the absence of extrapyramidal side effects at clinically effective doses. Nevertheless, despite years of research several important questions remain unanswered, foremost being the mechanisms whereby these drugs achieve their anti-'psychotic' effects. Patients suffering from schizophrenia are frequently reassured by their physicians that an antipsychotic drug will help clear the 'chemical imbalance'. While this chemical imbalance model is quite widely used and accepted by patients, we do not have a conceptual framework which addresses the complex issue of how a drug, essentially a pharmacological agent that effects change in a biological system, changes the personal experience of the patient. In this chapter we argue that not only is the modulation of dopaminergic neurotransmission key to the pharmacological action of antipsychotics, but it is also central to the understanding of the psychological mechanisms involved in the resolution of psychotic symptoms during antipsychotic treatment. The chapter draws heavily upon several previous articles by the first author.[7-10] In the interest of succinctness, the reader will be referred to these articles for further discussion and primary references relevant to the respective sections below.

The discussion will start with an outline of the empirical evidence for the relation between alteration in dopamine function and both antipsychotic drug action as well as the psychotic experience itself. We then discuss the involvement of dopamine as a mediator of motivational salience, a psychological construct referring to the involvement of dopamine in mediating the conversion of neutral information into meaningful stimuli that have the potential to influence goal-directed behaviour. Within this framework, psychotic symptoms are derived from aberrant attribution of meaning (or 'salience') to neutral stimuli, and the anti-psychotic effects of antipsychotic medications resulting from a 'dampening' of this aberrant salience through their actions on the mesolimbic dopaminergic system (Figure 14.1). Finally, the implications of this hypothesis for future research will be discussed.

Dopamine, psychosis and antipsychotics

The story of dopamine and psychosis is closely linked to its involvement in the mechanism of action of antipsychotic drugs, and the two have historically been subsumed under the umbrella of the dopamine hypothesis of schizophrenia.[11-13] Nonetheless, the evidence for dopamine's involvement in psychosis and antipsychotic drug action stems from two separate lines of research.

The lasting theories regarding the mechanism of action of antipsychotics were introduced by Carlsson and Lindquist, who showed that haloperidol and chlorpromazine increased the turnover of monoamines as reflected by increased levels of their metabolites,[14] and suggested that this effect might be compensatory to the drugs' blocking monoamine receptors. This finding led van Rossum[15] to postulate that antipsychotics might actually work via their action on dopamine receptors, although it was not until the work by Seeman and colleagues (and parallel findings by Synder and colleagues) that these receptors were actually identified and firmly linked to antipsychotic

---

Figure 14.1 (opposite) *The formation of delusional thinking through aberrant attribution of salience to neutral stimuli, and the effects of antipsychotics on both aberrant and normative saliences.*

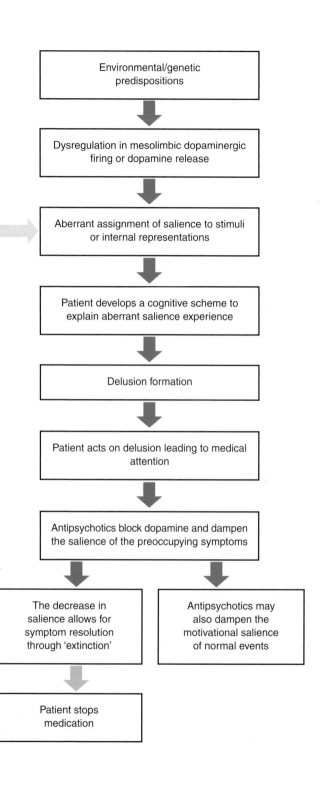

response.[16-19] All known antipsychotic medications, including atypical antipsychotic medications, bind to dopamine D_2 receptors. Positron emission tomography (PET) studies have shown that for most antipsychotics, the likelihood of clinical response is higher when at least 60% of central D_2 receptors are occupied by the drug, while extrapyramidal side effects (EPS) tend to occur when the D_2 receptor occupancy exceeds 80%.[20-26] Clozapine and quetiapine are effective antipsychotics at lower D_2-receptor occupancy, while aripiprazole, a partial dopamine D_2 receptor agonist, is effective at higher than 80% dopamine D_2 receptor occupancy in the absence of EPS – the significance and implications for this departure from the general rule are discussed elsewhere.[7,9,25,27–30]

Early evidence of a role for dopamine in psychosis stems largely from the effects of psychostimulants[31–35] which are known to induce psychotic experiences both in patients with schizophrenia as well as otherwise healthy subjects. Neuropathological abnormalities of dopaminergic indices obtained from post-mortem data in patients suffering from schizophrenia support this theory, although the interpretation of these data is confounded by previous antipsychotic treatment.[11,13] The most compelling evidence for the involvement of dopamine in psychosis comes from neuroimaging studies (details reviewed in references 12, 36, 37) which show increased dopamine synthesis,[38–41] an exaggerated release of dopamine,[42–44] and higher than normal levels of dopamine at baseline when psychotic[45,46] and some conflicting suggestions regarding an increase in receptor number.[47–51] Taken together these data support the central tenet of the dopamine hypothesis of schizophrenia, that is, the presence of a heightened dopaminergic transmission. This does not imply that dopaminergic dysregulation is the fundamental aspect of the pathophysiology of schizophrenia. On the contrary, it is more likely a 'state' abnormality associated with the dimension of positive psychotic symptoms of schizophrenia.

Why are antipsychotics anti-'psychotic'?

There is near-universal agreement for a central role of dopamine in 'reward' and 'motivation', although exactly what is meant by these terms is a matter of debate. There are a number of different theories that have been proposed to link dopamine to reward/motivation – and a number of different authors have tried to clarify the meaning of reward and motivation.[52–59] These theories share much in common and their differences are subtle to outsiders.

One of the more comprehensive accounts is the position of Berridge and Robinson[60,61] who suggest that one of the functional roles of dopamine is to mediate the conversion of an external stimulus from a neutral or 'cold bit' of sensory information into an 'attractive' and wanted entity or an 'aversive' and avoided entity.[60,62] In particular, the mesolimbic dopamine system is thought to be critical for the 'attribution of salience', a process whereby stimuli, events and perhaps even thoughts come to grab one's attention, drive action and influence goal-directed behaviour as a consequence of their association with reward or punishment.[60,62] This theory improves on the earlier hypothesis by Wise et al,[59,63,64] whereby dopamine is seen as a mediator of 'life's pleasures', irrespective of whether these are unconditioned stimuli such as food or sexual activity, or conditioned responses to neutral stimuli associated with them. In contrast to the theory of motivational salience, Wise et al's 'anhedonia hypothesis',[65] as it is commonly known, neither accounts for dopamine's mediation of unpleasurable stimuli (such as pain), nor the observation that firing of dopamine neurones actually precedes the rewarding or aversive experience (as though it were mediating some anticipatory or predictive function).

Normally, an external stimulus (e.g. a bright red brand new sports car speeding past a busy intersection) might result in a surge of dopamine in the mesolimbic system to mediate the acquisition and expression of appropriate motivational salience (e.g. pedestrian notices the car and turns to look at it) depending on one's experiences and predispositions (e.g. the pedestrian is an automobile enthusiast).[60,62,66,67] It should be noted that all aspects of this process are necessary components for the acquisition and expression of motivational salience (e.g. another pedestrian with no particular interest in cars might not have given the speeding car a second thought). Furthermore, dopamine functions as a 'mediator' rather than a 'creator' of salience in this process.

It is proposed that in psychosis a dysregulated dopamine transmission leads to a stimulus-inappropriate release of dopamine, that is, a normally neutral stimulus results in the firing of neurones in the mesolimbic system. This neurochemical aberration usurps the normal process of salience attribution, leading to aberrant assignment of salience to external objects or internal representations. Thus dopamine, which under normal conditions is a mediator of contextually relevant salience, in the psychotic state becomes a creator of salience, albeit an aberrant one.[10] The dopamine system normally attributes priority to novel situations, be they rewarding or aversive in nature, and that this attribution of salience is based on past experience and predispositions. It is proposed that in the earliest stages of the illness (i.e. during the prodrome) there is an exaggerated release of dopamine in the mesolimbic system that occurs out of context and independent of (that is, not causally related to) the situation. As a result, dopamine rather than 'mediating' salience of contextually and psychodynamically relevant stimuli and events, leads to the creation of aberrant salience and meaningfulness of otherwise neutral stimuli. This stage is often associated clinically with a sense of anxiety or confusion, which is followed by an intense need to make sense of the new realities being experienced (e.g. 'Why are the red cars driving by me all the time . . .'). It is proposed that the patient struggles with these aberrantly salient experiences and looks for meaning and explanation – often experiencing a sense of subjective relief and reduced perplexity as the delusion crystallizes ('the red colour means that I am going to come to harm . . .'). What is unique about the formation of these aberrant saliences is that unlike temporary distractions, they persist notwithstanding the absence of a sustained stimulus (clinicians often refer to this as a delusion 'taking a life of its own').

Thus, in this framework a delusion is a 'top-down' cognitive explanation that an individual imposes upon these aberrant salience experiences in an effort to make sense of them, and is by necessity imbued with the personal psychodynamic themes and embedded within an individual's cultural context. Standing on the same street with the zooming red car, another patient with a similar pathology may barely notice the car, but may become preoccupied by the passing cyclist glancing over his shoulder. The point here is that dopamine (or for that matter any chemical) cannot determine the content of the psychotic experience – it merely determines the underlying process. Such a dualist origin may explain why practitioners of psychodynamic psychotherapy have claimed that positive outcomes sometimes followed the 'analysis' of such psychotic experiences, even while cautioning that it has the potential for worsening of psychotic symptoms (presumably through the attribution of further salience to the psychotic experience of a perceived sustained stimulus).

Within the same framework, hallucinations arise from a conceptually similar but more direct process: the abnormal salience of internal representations of perceptions and memories leads to the subjective experience of these internal representations in a manner that is vivid and real, such that one is led to mistake this internal (virtual) experience with that of an external reality. In other words it is as though an individual is so engrossed by an internal (e.g. visual) representation of a thought or memory, that it is perceived with such intensity as though it were real. Thus, depending upon the salience devoted to an internal perception, an individual might perceive an auditory hallucination ranging from one's thoughts being heard within one's head all the way through a number of 'voices' heard outside one's head commenting on the patient's behaviour. In contrast to a categorical approach, this dimensional approach may explain experience of aberrant saliences ranging from the so called 'normal' – 'I thought I heard someone calling my name', to the 'expected' bereavement reaction of 'hearing' one's loved one, to the 'pathological' experience of auditory hallucinations experienced by patients suffering from schizophrenia.

It is proposed that antipsychotics are efficacious in psychosis because, by their pharmacological actions (involving the mesolimbic dopaminergic system at some level) they 'dampen salience' of the subjective experience of delusions and hallucinations. In this scheme, antipsychotics allow for the process of symptomatic improvement through further psychological and cognitive resolution by providing a platform of dampened salience. In doing so they do not change thoughts or ideas primarily, but provide a neurochemical milieu wherein previously acquired aberrant salience experiences are more likely to extinguish and new aberrant salience experiences are less likely to form.[68-70] This is consistent with how patients experience their symptomatic improvement following antipsychotic treatment: they do not immediately abandon the psychotic ideas or percepts, but report that the idea or percept 'doesn't bother me as much'.[71,72] While some patients do actually achieve complete resolution of their delusions and hallucinations with antipsychotic treatment, for most patients a dampening of symptoms is as good a resolution as antipsychotics can provide. At the same time as dampening the salience of symptoms, some normal-life saliences may also get dampened, perhaps leading to what is often called neuroleptic-induced dysphoria or drug-induced negative/depressive symptoms.

A theory of antipsychotic action must account not only for resolution of an acute psychotic episode, but also for the frequent observation of 'breakthrough' symptoms in patients maintained on antipsychotics, as well as full-blown relapses irrespective of whether the patient continues to be adherent to prescribed antipsychotic medication or in the common clinical scenario of discontinuation of medication. This model proposes that while the aberrant saliences are often dampened by the antipsychotic drug, they are not necessarily extinguished. Thus a surge of dopaminergic transmission (e.g. induced by a novel stressful situation or the use of psychostimulants or perhaps just a breakthrough in the putative neurochemical abnormality) or the removal of the antipsychotic would be expected to result in the emergence of symptoms that are similar if not the same in their theme as those experienced in the prior episodes.

Implications and future directions

The principal value of the model described above is the integration of the biological, pharmacological and psychodynamic factors that are involved in the response to antipsychotic drug treatment within one coherent framework. It does not, however, purport to explain any of the processes at work within the respective realms, nor does it impose limitations to the input functions at any of these levels. Thus, for example, while action of antipsychotics at the level of the mesolimbic dopaminergic system is proposed to mediate the dampening of aberrant saliences, this model does not exclude contributions from other mechanisms including serotonergic modulation of prefrontal release of dopamine, glutaminergic abnormalities or other emergent neurochemical mechanisms that might be involved in schizophrenia and other psychotic disorders. Similarly, no assumption is made as to which psychological process or processes might be directly impacted by the dampening of salience. Indeed, the model provides a template of how changes in one or more of a number of pharmacological, biological or psychological factors might be expected to interact. Furthermore, the model predicts that dampening aberrant salience with antipsychotics needs to be accompanied by non-pharmacological interventions in order that the healing process involving cognitive and psychological restructuring might take place. While the onset of this healing process might be expected to be immediate, the disavowal of aberrant saliences might be expected to be both lengthy and possibly incomplete.

This model also predicts that antipsychotic drugs, by virtue of dampening motivational salience, result in the unwanted dampening of other saliences for objects and ideas that one loves or desires. Since these saliences drive us to expend time and energy in activities such as interpersonal relationships and occupational or recreational pursuits, it is quite conceivable (and indeed consistent with clinical experience) that antipsychotics may take out some of the fire of life's normal motivations, desires and pleasures. This might account for previously described symptoms such as 'neuroleptic-induced dysphoria', an unpleasant subjective experience that differs from the subjective sensation of low mood. This does not imply that antipsychotics necessarily dampen normal and abnormal saliences to the same extent – more than likely this effect is asymmetrical – although it is unlikely that any one of the currently available antipsychotic drugs exclusively targets aberrant saliences while leaving the normative ones intact. In fact, the pre-clinical literature is replete with studies that demonstrate unequivocally the impact of antipsychotics on normal motivational drives (e.g. Wise et al[59] and Wise and Colle[64]).

Finally, the model is one of psychosis, or more specifically delusions and perhaps hallucinations. It neither purports to account for the pathophysi-ology of schizophrenia, nor does it include other important manifestations of this disorder such as affective and negative symptoms, which in fact show limited response to the current generation(s) of antipsychotic drugs.

'All models are wrong, some models are useful' (attributed to a certain Deming). Given that the current model is based on empirical data related to dopamine, schizophrenia, and antipsychotics – evidence that is subject to ongoing revision with new research findings – the model is just a beginning. Rather than being presented in a form that leads to a single pivotal prediction, it provides a heuristic framework that may be used to bridge a number of empirical biological data with phenomenological reports and clinical observations. The basis of the model does, however, rest on, or at least make predictions about, a central role for dopamine in psy-chosis, about a process such as 'salience' being central to psychosis, about psychosis being an interactive product of the mind and the brain and about antipsychotics dampening psychosis rather than excising it. It is hoped that as more knowledge is accrued in each of these areas, the model will be revised bringing it closer to the true processes and their interactions that lead to the experience of psychosis, the mechanism whereby antipsychotics contribute the process of healing, as well as the healing process itself. Time will tell whether this is a realistic goal or just an aberrantly salient idea har-boured by the authors.

Acknowledgements

Dr Kapur is supported by a Canada Research Chair. Dr Mamo is supported by the Cleghorn Fellowship at the University of Toronto.

References

1. Frankenburg FR, History of the development of antipsychotic medication. *Psychiatr Clin North Am* 1994; **17**:531–540.
2. Healy D, *The Creation of Psychopharmacology*. Harvard University Press: Cambridge, MA, 2002.
3. Delay J, Deniker P, Harl J, Traitment des etats d'excitation et d'agitation par une methode medicamenteuse derivée de l'hibernotherapie. *Ann Med Psychol* 1952; **110**:267–273.
4. Kline N, Use of *Rauwolfia serpentina* in neuropsychiatric conditions. *Ann NY Acad Sci* 1955; **61**:107–132.
5. Hollister L, Krieger G, Kringel A, Roberts R, Treatment of schizophrenia reactions with reserpine. *Ann NY Acad Sci* 1955; **61**:92–100.
6. King C, Voruganti LN, What's in a name? The evolution of the nomenclature of antipsychotic drugs. *J Psychiatry Neurosci* 2002; **27**:168–175.
7. Kapur S, Remington G, Dopamine D(2) receptors and their role in atypical antipsychotic action: still necessary and may even be sufficient. *Biol Psychiatry* 2001; **50**:873–883.
8. Kapur S, Remington G, Atypical antipsychotics: new directions and new challenges in the treatment of schizophrenia. *Annu Rev Med* 2001; **52**:503–517.
9. Kapur S, Seeman P, Does fast dissociation from the dopamine D(2) receptor explain the action of atypical antipsychotics?: A new hypothesis. *Am J Psychiatry* 2001; **158**:360–369.
10. Kapur S, Psychosis as a state of aberrant salience: a framework linking biology, phenomenology, and pharmacology in schizophrenia. *Am J Psychiatry* 2003; **160**:13–23.
11. Seeman P, Dopamine receptors and the dopamine hypothesis of schizophrenia. *Synapse* 1987; **1**:133–152.
12. Seeman P, Kapur S, Schizophrenia: more dopamine, more D2 receptors. *Proc Natl Acad Sci USA* 2000; **97**:7673–7675.
13. Davis KL, Kahn RS, Ko G, Davidson M, Dopamine in schizophrenia: a review and reconceptualization. *Am J Psychiatry* 1991; **148**:1474–1486.
14. Carlsson A, Lindquist M, Effect of chlorpromazine or haloperidol on the formation of 3-methoxytyramine and normetanephrine in mouse brain. *Acta Pharmacol Toxicol* 1963; **20**:140–144.
15. van Rossum J, The significance of dopamine-receptor blockade for the action of neuroleptic drugs. In: Bradley P (ed). *Neuropsychopharmacology, Proceedings 5th Collegium Internationale Neuropsychopharmacologicum* pp. 321–329 Excerpta Medica: Amsterdam, 1967.
16. Seeman P, Chau-Wong M, Tedesco J, Wong K, Brain receptors for antipsychotic drugs and dopamine: direct binding assays. *Proc Natl Acad Sci USA* 1975; **72**:4376–4380.
17. Seeman P, Lee T, Antipsychotic drugs: direct correlation between clinical potency and presynaptic action on dopamine neurons. *Science* 1975; **188**:1217–1219.
18. Seeman P, Lee T, Chau-Wong M, Wong K, Antipsychotic drug doses and neuroleptic/dopamine receptors. *Nature* 1976; **261**:717–719.
19. Creese I, Burt DR, Snyder SH, Dopamine receptor binding predicts clinical and pharmacological potencies of antischizophrenic drugs. *Science* 1976; **192**:481–483.
20. Farde L, Nordstrom AL, Wiesel FA, Pauli S, Halldin C, Sedvall G, Positron emission tomographic analysis of central D1 and D2 dopamine receptor occupancy in patients treated with classical neuroleptics and clozapine. Relation to extrapyramidal side effects. *Arch Gen Psychiatry* 1992; **49**:538–544.
21. Nordstrom AL, Farde L, Wiesel FA et al, Central D2-dopamine receptor occupancy

in relation to antipsychotic drug effects: a double-blind PET study of schizophrenic patients. *Biol Psychiatry* 1993; **33**:227–235.

22. Kapur S, Zipursky R, Jones C, Remington G, Houle S, Relationship between dopamine D(2) occupancy, clinical response, and side effects: a double-blind PET study of first-episode schizophrenia. *Am J Psychiatry* 2000; **157**:514–520.

23. Nyberg S, Farde L, Halldin C, A PET study of 5-HT2 and D2 dopamine receptor occupancy induced by olanzapine in healthy subjects. *Neuropsychopharmacology* 1997; **16**:1–7.

24. Kapur S, Zipursky RB, Jones C et al, The D2 receptor occupancy profile of loxapine determined using PET. *Neuropsychopharmacology* 1996; **15**:562–566.

25. Kapur S, Zipursky RB, Remington G, Clinical and theoretical implications of 5-HT2 and D2 receptor occupancy of clozapine, risperidone, and olanzapine in schizophrenia. *Am J Psychiatry* 1999; **156**:286–293.

26. Kapur S, Zipursky RB, Remington G et al, 5-HT2 and D2 receptor occupancy of olanzapine in schizophrenia: a PET investigation. *Am J Psychiatry* 1998; **155**:921–928.

27. Kane JM, Carson WH, Saha AR et al, Efficacy and safety of aripiprazole and haloperidol versus placebo in patients with schizophrenia and schizoaffective disorder. *J Clin Psychiatry* 2002; **63**:763–771.

28. Lawler CP, Prioleau C, Lewis MM et al, Interactions of the novel antipsychotic aripiprazole (OPC-14597) with dopamine and serotonin receptor subtypes. *Neuropsychopharmacology* 1999; **20**:612–627.

29. Burris KD, Molski TF, Xu C et al, Aripiprazole, a novel antipsychotic, is a high-affinity partial agonist at human dopamine D2 receptors. *J Pharmacol Exp Ther* 2002; **302**:381–389.

30. Kapur S, Zipursky R, Jones C, Shammi CS, Remington G, Seeman P, A positron emission tomography study of quetiapine in schizophrenia: a preliminary finding of an antipsychotic effect with only transiently high dopamine D2 receptor occupancy. *Arch Gen Psychiatry* 2000; **57**:553–559.

31. Harris D, Batki SL, Stimulant psychosis: symptom profile and acute clinical course. *Am J Addict* 2000; **9**:28–37.

32. Angrist B, Lee HK, Gershon S, The antagonism of amphetamine-induced symptomatology by a neuroleptic. *Am J Psychiatry* 1974; **131**:817–819.

33. Angrist B, Rotrosen J, Gershon S, Responses to apomorphine, amphetamine, and neuroleptics in schizophrenic subjects. *Psychopharmacology (Berl)* 1980; **67**:31–38.

34. Angrist B, Sathananthan G, Wilk S, Gershon S, Amphetamine psychosis: behavioral and biochemical aspects. *J Psychiatr Res* 1974; **11**:13–23.

35. Angrist BM, Gershon S, The phenomenology of experimentally induced amphetamine psychosis – preliminary observations. *Biol Psychiatry* 1970; **2**:95–107.

36. Soares JC, Innis RB, Neurochemical brain imaging investigations of schizophrenia. *Biol Psychiatry* 1999; **46**:600–615.

37. Laruelle M, Abi-Dargham A, Dopamine as the wind of the psychotic fire: new evidence from brain imaging studies. *J Psychopharmacol* 1999; **13**:358–371.

38. Reith J, Benkelfat C, Sherwin A et al, Elevated dopa decarboxylase activity in living brain of patients with psychosis. *Proc Nat Acad Sci USA* 1994; **91**:11651–11654.

39. Hietala J, Syvalahti E, Vuorio K et al, Presynaptic dopamine function in striatum of neuroleptic-naive schizophrenic patients. *Lancet* 1995; **346**:1130–1131.

40. Meyer-Lindenberg A, Miletich RS, Kohn PD et al, Reduced prefrontal activity predicts exaggerated striatal dopaminergic function in schizophrenia. *Nat Neurosci* 2002; **5**:267–271.

41. Lindstrom LH, Gefvert O, Hagberg G et al, Increased dopamine synthesis rate in medial prefrontal cortex and striatum in schizophrenia indicated by L-(beta-11C) DOPA and PET. *Biol Psychiatry* 1999; **46**:681–688.

42. Laruelle M, Abi-Dargham A, van Dyck CH et al, Single photon emission computerized tomography imaging of amphetamine-induced dopamine release in drug-free schizophrenic subjects. *Proc Natl Acad Sci USA* 1996; **93**:9235–9240.

43. Abi-Dargham A, Gil R, Krystal J et al, Increased striatal dopamine transmission in schizophrenia: confirmation in a second cohort. *Am J Psychiatry* 1998; **155**:761–767.

44. Breier A, Su TP, Saunders R et al, Schizophrenia is associated with elevated amphetamine-induced synaptic dopamine concentrations: evidence from a novel positron emission tomography method. *Proc Natl Acad Sci USA* 1997; **94**:2569–2574.

45. Abi-Dargham A, Rodenhiser J, Printz D et al, From the cover: increased baseline occupancy of D2 receptors by dopamine in schizophrenia. *Proc Natl Acad Sci USA* 2000; **97**:8104–8109.

46. Gjedde A, Wong DF, Quantification of neuroreceptors in living human brain. v. endogenous neurotransmitter inhibition of haloperidol binding in psychosis. *J Cereb Blood Flow Metab* 2001; **21**:982–994.

47. Wong DF, Wagner HN Jr, Tune L et al, Positron emission tomography reveals elevated D_2 dopamine receptors in drug-naive schizophrenics. *Science* 1986; **234**:1558–1563.

48. Wong DF, Pearlson GD, Tune LE et al, Quantification of neuroreceptors in the living human brain. 4. Effect of aging and elevations of D-2-like receptors in schizophrenia and bipolar illness. *J Cereb Blood Flow Metab* 1997; **17**:331–342.

49. Andreasen NC, Carson R, Diksic M et al, Workshop on schizophrenia, PET, and dopamine D_2 receptors in the human neostriatum. *Schizophr Bull* 1988; **14**:471–484.

50. Farde L, Wiesel FA, Stone-Elander S et al, D2 dopamine receptors in neuroleptic-naive schizophrenic patients. *Arch Gen Psychiatry* 1990; **47**:213–219.

51. Nordstrom AL, Farde L, Eriksson L, Halldin C, No elevated d-2 dopamine receptors in neuroleptic-naive schizophrenic patients revealed by positron emission tomography and [c-11]n-methylspiperone. *Psychiatry Res Neuroimag* 1995; **61**:67–83.

52. Salamone JD, Cousins MS, Snyder BJ, Behavioral functions of nucleus accumbens dopamine: empirical and conceptual problems with the anhedonia hypothesis. *Neurosci Biobehav Rev* 1997; **21**:341–359.

53. Robbins TW, Everitt BJ, Neurobehavioural mechanisms of reward and motivation. *Curr Opin Neurobiol* 1996; **6**:228–236.

54. Horvitz JC, Mesolimbocortical and nigrostriatal dopamine responses to salient non-reward events. *Neuroscience* 2000; **96**:651–656.

55. Bindra D, A motivational view of learning, performance, and behavior modification. *Psychol Rev* 1974; **81**:199–213.

56. Di Chiara G, A motivational learning hypothesis of the role of mesolimbic dopamine in compulsive drug use. *J Psychopharmacol* 1998; **12**:54–67.

57. Toates F, The interaction of cognitive and stimulus-response processes in the control of behaviour. *Neurosci Biobehav Rev* 1998; **22**:59–83.

58. Fibiger HC, Phillips AG, Mesocorticolimbic dopamine systems and reward. *Ann NY Acad Sci* 1988; **537**:206–215.

59. Wise RA, Spindler J, deWit H, Gerberg GJ, Neuroleptic-induced 'anhedonia' in rats: pimozide blocks reward quality of food. *Science* 1978; **201**:262–264.

60. Berridge KC, Robinson TE, What is the role of dopamine in reward: hedonic impact, reward learning, or incentive salience? *Brain Res Brain Res Rev* 1998; **28**:309–369.

61. Berridge KC, Robinson TE, Parsing reward. *Trends Neurosci* 2003; **26**:507–513.

62. Berridge KC, Pleasure, pain, desire and dread: hidden core processes of emotion. In: Schwarz N (ed), *Well Being: The Foundations of Hedonic Psychology*. Russel Sage Foundation: New York, 1999.

63. Wise RA, Neuroleptic attenuation of intracranial self-stimulation: reward or performance deficits? *Life Sci* 1978; **22**:535–42.

64. Wise RA, Colle LM, Pimozide attenuates free feeding: best scores analysis reveals a motivational deficit. *Psychopharmacology (Berl)* 1984; **84**:446–451.

65. Wise R. Neuroleptics and operant behavior: the anhedonia hypothesis. *Behav Brain Sci* 1982; **5**:39–87.

66. Shizgal P, Neural basis of utility estimation. *Curr Opin Neurobiol* 1997; **7**:198–208.

67. Heinz A, [Anhedonia – a general nosology surmounting correlate of a dysfunctional dopaminergic reward system?]. *Nervenarzt* 1999; **70**:391–398.

68. Clody DE, Carlton PL, Stimulus efficacy, chlorpromazine, and schizophrenia. *Psychopharmacology* 1980; **69**:127–131.

69. Miller R, The time course of neuroleptic therapy for psychosis: role of learning processes and implications for concepts of psychotic illness. *Psychopharmacology* 1987; **92**:405–415.

70. Miller R, Hyperactivity of associations in psychosis. *Aust NZ J Psychiatry* 1989; **23**:241–248.

71. Winkelman NW, Chlorpromazine in the treament of neuropsychiatric disorders. *JAMA* 1954; **155**:18–21.

72. Elkes J, Elkes C, Effect of chlorpromazine on the behaviour of chronically overactive psychotic patients. *BMJ* 1954; **2**:560–565.

chapter 15

'Gone to pot': pharmacological evidence supporting the contribution of cannabinoid receptor function to psychosis

D Cyril D'Souza

The association between cannabis and psychosis is not a new one. It was described as far back as 1845 that use of hashish was associated with acute psychotic reactions that sometimes could last up to days.[1] Since then several other studies support an association between cannabis and psychosis (reviewed in reference 2). However, the precise nature of the association remains unclear. The existing literature is based mainly on naturalistic studies. These data have limitations including inadequate patient selection and sample size, poorly defined inclusion criteria, absence of standardized assessments, a reliance on self-report of psychosis, lack of a urine toxicology to confirm cannabis use and exclude other drug use, and crude information about dose–response relations. Most importantly, some naturalistic studies cannot, because of their retrospective nature, confirm the psychiatric health status of individuals who later go on to develop psychosis. Some of these limitations can be addressed in laboratory studies.

Several studies suggest that cannabis is among the most frequently used illicit substances by patients with schizophrenia.[3–10] However, little is known about why these patients use cannabis or what effects cannabis has on the symptoms associated with schizophrenia. Several studies suggest that patients with schizophrenia may use cannabis to relieve or 'self-medicate' symptoms,[11–17] side effects,[18] to relieve boredom, to 'get high', or to 'relax' and to socialize with peers.[7,14,18,19] In contrast, epidemiological data suggest that cannabis use has a negative impact on the expression and course of schizophrenia.[16,20–26] However, the existing literature is based on retrospective self-report data which are subject to distortion. Therefore we performed a controlled laboratory study to investigate the impact of Δ-9-tetrahydracannabinol (Δ-9-THC) on symptomatology and cognitive functioning in patients with schizophrenia and healthy controls.

Methods

In a 3-day, double blind, randomized and counterbalanced study, the behavioural, cognitive, motor and endocrine effects of 0, 2.5 mg and 5 mg intravenous Δ-9-THC were characterized in stable, antipsychotic-treated schizophrenia or schizo-affective disorder patients (n = 13). Healthy controls (n = 22) carefully screened for any obvious family history of psychosis or any risk for developing psychosis were studied in parallel. Only individuals with exposure to cannabis but without a lifetime history of cannabis abuse disorder were studied. Cannabis-naive individuals were excluded in order to minimize the risk of subjects becoming addicted to cannabis after participating in the study.

The consent process involved several documented sessions and included an ombudsperson. Understanding of the study was confirmed using a questionnaire. There were clear stopping rules specified a priori with provisions for rescue medications and hospitalization. Prospective safety data at 1, 3 and 6 months post-study were collected to determine whether exposure to Δ-9-THC in the laboratory had any impact in the short or long term on schizophrenia and future cannabis use.

The three test days were at least 7 days apart to account for the long half-life of Δ-9-THC. Δ-9-THC was administered intravenously to avoid the substantial inter- and intraindividual variation in delivery of Δ-9-THC with the inhaled route. Data were analysed in SAS PROC MIXED using mixed effects models with dose (placebo, 2.5 mg and 5 mg), time (P10, P80, P200) and the dose by time interaction as fixed effects and structured variance–covariance pattern matrix.

Effects of Δ-9-THC in schizophrenia patients and healthy controls

Δ-9-THC increased scores of the PANSS (Positive and Negative Syndrome Scale) positive symptoms subscale in the patients with schizophrenia. The increases in positive symptoms were modest and by the last time point, positive symptoms returned to baseline levels (Figure 15.1). The positive symptoms reported to increase were generally those symptoms that were unique to their individual condition.

Δ-9-THC also transiently increased scores of the PANSS positive symptoms subscale in healthy controls. The increases in positive symptoms were modest and by the last time point, positive symptom scores returned to baseline levels. Some of the positive symptoms reported by healthy subjects were similar to positive symptoms of the schizophrenic patients including suspiciousness, grandiosity, conceptual disorganization and unusual thought content. For example, one healthy subject reported that research staff were

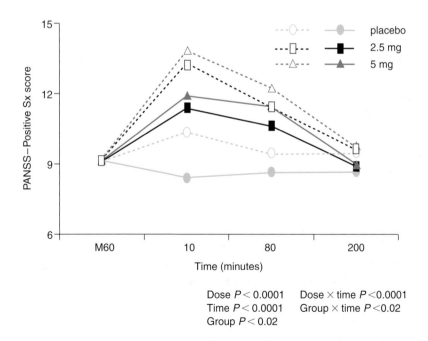

Figure 15.1 *Effect of Δ-9-THC on the positive symptoms (Sx) subscale of the Positive and Negative Syndrome Scale (PANSS) in healthy controls (———) and patients with schizophrenia (– – – –).*

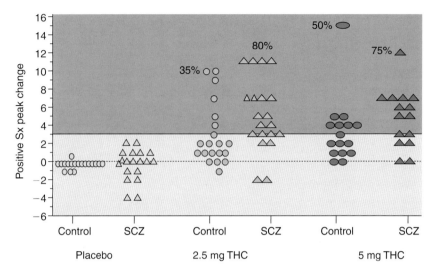

Figure 15.2 *Peak increases in positive symptoms (Sx) in healthy controls and patients with schizophrenia (SCZ) following administration of placebo, 2.5 mg and 5 mg of Δ-9-THC.*

trying to trick her by changing the rules of some of the cognitive tests, while another reported that he thought that research staff were surreptitiously administering Δ-9-THC through the blood pressure machine and the sheets (suspiciousness). Other subjects reported not being able to keep track of their thoughts, or that their thoughts were occurring in staccato (conceptual disorganization) and feeling that everything was happening all at once and that their thoughts were fragmented. Some healthy subjects reported feeling that research staff could read their minds, or that they felt they could look into the future (unusual thought content).

In a preliminary analysis, the effects of Δ-9-THC on clinically significant positive symptoms were compared in the two groups (Figure 15.2). Clinically significant positive symptoms were defined as an increase of three or more points on the positive symptom scale of the PANSS. A greater proportion of schizophrenic patients experienced clinically significant psychosis relative to healthy subjects. Δ-9-THC also significantly increased perceptual alterations measured by the Clinician Administered Dissociative Symptoms Scale in a dose-dependent manner in both groups.

Δ-9-THC significantly increased negative symptoms measured by the negative symptoms subscale of the PANSS (Figure 15.3). However, the known sedating and cataleptic effects of Δ-9-THC may have confounded the

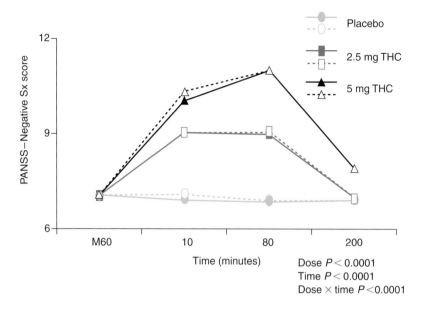

Figure 15.3 *Δ-9-THC –induced negative symptoms (Sx) measured by the negative symptoms subscale of the Positive and Negative Syndrome Scale (PANSS) in healthy controls (————) and patients with schizophrenia (– – – –).*

assessment of negative symptoms. Further, challenge studies are not the best way of actually evaluating negative symptoms. Nevertheless, these were statistically significant results (see Figure 15.3).

Δ-9-THC reduced immediate recall in healthy subjects and in schizophrenic patients (Figure 15.4). At the 5 mg dose of Δ-9-THC, the immediate recall performance of healthy controls was the same as that of schizophrenic patients on the placebo day. Schizophrenic patients appeared to be more sensitive to the effects of Δ-9-THC on immediate recall. Similarly, Δ-9-THC also disrupted delayed recall in a statistically significant manner (see Figure 15.4) but there were no obvious differences between controls and schizophrenic patients.

The participants were contacted 1, 3, 6 and 9 months after the study. In neither group was there evidence to suggest that exposure to Δ-9-THC in the study had a negative impact on future cannabis use. In schizophrenic patients, there was no evidence to suggest that participation had a negative impact on the long- or short-term course of schizophrenia (hospitalization rate, emergency rooms visits, etc.).

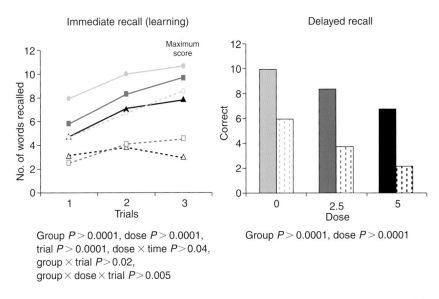

Group $P > 0.0001$, dose $P > 0.0001$,
trial $P > 0.0001$, dose $\times$ time $P > 0.04$,
group $\times$ trial $P > 0.02$,
group $\times$ dose $\times$ trial $P > 0.005$

Group $P > 0.0001$, dose $P > 0.0001$

Figure 15.4 Δ-9-THC-impaired learning in healthy controls (———) and patients with schizophrenia (– – – –); Δ-9-THC-impaired memory (delayed recall) in controls (solid bars) and patients with schizophrenia (patterned bars).

In summary, Δ-9-THC transiently exacerbated symptoms in schizophrenic patients and induced a spectrum of schizophrenia-like symptoms in healthy controls. There were no 'beneficial' effects of Δ-9-THC on either the symptoms or the side effects associated with schizophrenia. Group differences in vulnerability to Δ-9-THC were perhaps masked by the fact that only clinically stable schizophrenic patients, all taking dopamine D_2 antagonists, were studied. The mechanism by which Δ-9-THC exacerbated symptoms in schizophrenic patients and induced psychotic symptoms in healthy subjects is not known and warrants further study.

Cannabinoids, dopamine and psychosis

Among the candidate mechanisms are dopaminergic mechanisms by which cannabinoids produce psychosis. Behavioural, biochemical and electrophysiological data demonstrate the involvement of dopaminergic systems in some of the actions of cannabinoids. Δ-9-THC has been shown to enhance neuronal firing of mesolimbic dopamine projections from ventral tegmental area (VTA) to nucleus accumbens (NAc).[27–29] Δ-9-THC has also been shown to increase the release of dopamine in the shell of the NAc,[30–32] an effect that is also seen with heroin, cocaine, D-amphetamine and nicotine. Of note is that the effects of Δ-9-THC on fos expression are blocked by dopamine antagonists.[33] Consistent with electrophysiological studies, CB-1R agonists induce cfos in the NAc[33] and A10 dopaminergic neurones within the VTA[34] and these effects are blocked by dopamine D_2 receptor antagonists[33] and CB-1R antagonists.[34,35]

If dopaminergic systems play an important role in Δ-9-THC psychosis then dopamine D_2 antagonists might block these effects. The second ongoing project aimed at evaluating the effects of haloperidol on the Δ-9-THC response in a double blind, randomized, placebo-controlled study of healthy subjects. Only subjects with exposure to cannabis but without a lifetime history of cannabis abuse disorder were studied. Cannabis-naive individuals were excluded in order to minimize the risk of subjects becoming addicted to cannabis after participating in the study. Healthy subjects received 0.05 mg/kg haloperidol (3.5 mg in a 70 kg individual) or placebo, and then a fixed order of placebo and Δ-9-THC (0.05 mg/kg) infusions. Thus, 90 minutes after receiving placebo or haloperidol, subjects received placebo Δ-9-THC, followed 120 minutes later by active Δ-9-THC.

As expected, Δ-9-THC (0.05 mg/kg) increased positive symptoms measured by the PANSS positive symptoms subscale. However, haloperidol had no effect on Δ-9-THC-induced psychotic symptoms (Figure 15.5). These preliminary findings suggest that dopamine D_2 receptor antagonists may not be

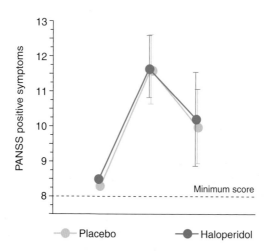

Figure 15.5 *Haloperidol does not reduce Δ-9-THC-induced positive symptoms measured by the Positive and Negative Syndrome Scale (PANSS).*

useful in Δ-9-THC-related psychosis and that dopaminergic systems may not play a major role in the psychotogenic effects of cannabinoids.

Δ-9-THC 'model' psychosis and implications for the neurobiology of psychoses

The amphetamine and the ketamine paradigms were critical in advancing the dopamine and glutamate hypothesis. The finding that Δ-9-THC induced transient positive, negative and cognitive symptoms in healthy people similar to those seen in schizophrenia is intriguing and suggests a cannabinoid hypothesis of psychosis. Data from converging lines of evidence provide tentative support for this hypothesis. The findings from the pharmacological study discussed in this chapter collectively with data from post-mortem,[36] epidemiological,[37–41] neurochemical[42] and genetic[43] studies warrant investigation of whether cannabinoid receptor system dysfunction contributes to the pathophysiology and treatment of schizophrenia.

Acknowledgements

National Institute of Mental Health (R01 MH61019-02 to DCD) National Institute of Drug Abuse (R01 DA12382-01 to DCD), Stanley Foundation (DCD), Donaghue Foundation (DCD).

References

1. Moreau de Tours J, Sobre el hachisch y la alienacion mental. *Actas Luso-Espanolas de Neurologia, Psiquiatria y Ciencias Afines* 1973; **1**:477–484.
2. Johns A, Psychiatric effects of cannabis. *Br J Psychiatry* 2001; **178**:116–122.
3. Mueser KT, Bellack AS, Blanchard JJ, Comorbidity of schizophrenia and substance abuse: implications for treatment. *J Consul Clin Psychol* 1992; **60**:845–856.
4. Cuffel BJ, Heithoff KA, Lawson W, Correlates of patterns of substance abuse among patients with schizophrenia. *Hospital Community Psychiatry* 1993; **44**:247–251.
5. Kessler RC, Foster CL, Saunders WB, Stang PE, Social consequences of psychiatric disorders, I: Educational attainment. *Am J Psychiatry* 1995; **152**:1026–1032.
6. Hambrecht M, Hafner H, Substance abuse and the onset of schizophrenia. *Biol Psychiatry* 1996; **40**:1155–1163.
7. Fowler IL, Carr VJ, Carter NT, Lewin TJ, Patterns of current and lifetime substance use in schizophrenia. *Schizophr Bull* 1998; **24**:443–455.
8. Farrell M, Howes S, Taylor C et al, Substance misuse and psychiatric comorbidity: an overview of the OPCS National Psychiatric Morbidity Survey. *Addict Behav* 1998; **23**:909–918.
9. Jablensky A, McGrath J, Herrman H et al, Psychotic disorders in urban areas: an

overview of the Study on Low Prevalence Disorders. *Aust NZ J Psychiatry* 2000; **34**:221–236.

10. Buhler B, Hambrecht M, Loffler W, an der Heiden W, Hafner H, Precipitation and determination of the onset and course of schizophrenia by substance abuse – a retrospective and prospective study of 232 population-based first illness episodes. *Schizophr Res* 2002; **54**:243–251.

11. Schneier FR, Siris SG, A review of psychoactive substance use and abuse in schizophrenia. Patterns of drug choice. *J Nerv Ment Dis* 1987; **175**:641–652.

12. Dixon L, Haas G, Weiden J, Sweeney J, Frances AJ, Drug abuse in schizophrenic patients: clinical correlates and reasons for use. *Am J Psychiatry* 1991; **148**: 224–230.

13. Peralta V, Cuesta MJ, Influence of cannabis abuse on schizophrenic psychopathology. *Acta Psychiatr Scand* 1992; **85**:127–130.

14. Addington J, Duchak V, Reasons for substance use in schizophrenia. *Acta Psychiatr Scand* 1997; **96**:329–333.

15. Addington J, Addington D, Substance abuse and cognitive functioning in schizophrenia.[Comment]. *J Psychiatry Neurosci* 1997; **22**:99–104.

16. Brunette MF, Mueser KT, Xie H, Drake RE, Relationships between symptoms of schizophrenia and substance abuse. *J Nerv Ment Dis* 1997; **185**:13–20.

17. Phillips P, Johnson S, How does drug and alcohol misuse develop among people with psychotic illness? A literature review. *Soc Psychiatry Psychiatr Epidemiol* 2001; **36**:269–276.

18. Dixon L, Haas G, Weiden P, Sweeney J, Frances A, Acute effects of drug abuse in schizophrenic patients: clinical observations and patients' self-reports. *Schizophr Bull* 1990; **16**:69–79.

19. Mueser KT, Yarnold PR, Bellack AS, Diagnostic and demographic correlates of substance abuse in schizophrenia and major affective disorder. *Acta Psychiatr Scand* 1992; **85**:48–55.

20. Negrete JC, Knapp WP, The effects of cannabis use on the clinical condition of schizophrenics. *NIDA Res Monogr* 1986; **67**:321–327.

21. Negrete JC, Knapp WP, Douglas DE, Smith WB, Cannabis affects the severity of schizophrenic symptoms: results of a clinical survey. *Psychol Med* 1986; **16**:515–20.

22. Linszen DH, Dingemans PM, Lenior ME, Cannabis abuse and the course of recent-onset schizophrenic disorders. *Arch Gen Psychiatry* 1994; **51**:273–9.

23. Caspari D, Cannabis and schizophrenia: results of a follow-up study. *Eur Arch Psychiatry Clin Neurosci* 1999; **249**:45–49.

24. Dixon L, Dual diagnosis of substance abuse in schizophrenia: prevalence and impact on outcomes. *Schizophr Res* 1999; **35(Suppl)**:S93–100.

25. Liraud F, Verdoux H, [Effect of comorbid substance use on neuropsychological performance in subjects with psychotic or mood disorders]. *Encephale* 2002; **28**:160–168.

26. Liraud F, Verdoux H, [Clinical and prognostic characteristics associated with addictive comorbidity in hospitalized psychiatric patients]. *Encephale* 2000; **26**:16–23.

27. French ED, delta9-tetrahydrocannabinol excites rat VTA dopamine neurons through activation of cannabinoid CB1 but not opioid receptors. *Neurosci Lett* 1997; **226**:159–162.

28. French ED, Dillon K, Wu X, Cannabinoids excite dopamine neurons in the ventral tegmentum and substantia nigra. *Neuroreport* 1997; **8**:649–652.

29. Melis M, Gessa GL, Diana M, Different mechanisms for dopaminergic excitation induced by opiates and cannabinoids in the rat midbrain. *Prog Neuropsychopharmacol Biol Psychiatry* 2000; **24**:993–1006.

30. Chen J, Paredes W, Lowinson JH, Gardner EL, Delta-9-tetrahydrocannabinol

enhances presynaptic dopamine efflux in medial prefrontal cortex. *Eur J Pharmacol* 1990; **190**:259–262.

31. Chen JP, Paredes W, Lowinson JH, Gardner EL, Strain-specific facilitation of dopamine efflux by delta-9-tetrahydrocannabinol in the nucleus accumbens of rat: an in vivo microdialysis study. *Neuroscience Letters* 1991; **129**:136–180.

32. Tanda G, Pontieri FE, Di Chiara G, Cannabinoid and heroin activation of mesolimbic dopamine transmission by a common mu1 opioid receptor mechanism. [Comment]. *Science* 1997; **276**:2048–2050.

33. Miyamoto A, Yamamoto T, Ohno M et al, Roles of dopamine D1 receptors in delta 9-tetrahydrocannabinol-induced expression of Fos protein in the rat brain. *Brain Res* 1996; **710**:234–240.

34. Patel S, Hillard CJ, Cannabinoid-induced Fos expression within A10 dopaminergic neurons. *Brain Res*, 2003; **963**:15–25.

35. Porcella A, Gessa GL, Pani L, Delta9-tetrahydrocannabinol increases sequence-specific AP-1 DNA-binding activity and Fos-related antigens in the rat brain. *Eur J Neurosci* 1998; **10**:1743–1751.

36. Dean B, Sundram S, Bradbury R, Scarr E, Copolov D, Studies on [3H]CP-55940 binding in the human central nervous system: regional specific changes in density of cannabinoid-1 receptors associated with schizophrenia and cannabis use. *Neuroscience* 2001; **103**:9–15.

37. Andreasson S, Allebeck P, Engstrom A, Rydberg U, Cannabis and schizophrenia. A longitudinal study of Swedish conscripts. *Lancet* 1987; **2**:1483–1486.

38. Zammit S, Allebeck P, Andreasson S, Lundberg I, Lewis G, Self reported cannabis use as a risk factor for schizophrenia in Swedish conscripts of 1969: historical cohort study. *BMJ* 2002; **325**:1199.

39. Andreasson S, Allebeck P, Engstrom A, Rydberg U, Cannabis and schizophrenia. *Lancet* 1988; **1**:1000–1001.

40. Arseneault L, Cannon M, Poulton R et al, Cannabis use in adolescence and risk for adult psychosis: longitudinal prospective study. *BMJ* 2002; **325**:1212–1213.

41. McGuire PK, Jones P, Harvey I et al, Morbid risk of schizophrenia for relatives of patients with cannabis-associated psychosis. *Schizophr Res* 1995; **15**:277–281.

42. Leweke FM, Giuffrida A, Wurster U, Emrich HM, Piomelli D, Elevated endogenous cannabinoids in schizophrenia. *Neuroreport* 1999; **10**:1665–1669.

43. Ujike H, Takaki M, Nakata K et al, CNR1, central cannabinoid receptor gene, associated with susceptibility to hebephrenic schizophrenia. *Mol Psychiatry* 2002; **7**:515–518.

chapter 16

Schizophrenia represents a failure to regulate dopamine systems

Anthony A Grace

One of the prominent hypotheses regarding the pathophysiology of schizophrenia is the dopamine hypothesis of schizophrenia. This model is based on several findings: (i) drugs that increase dopamine release in the brain, such as amphetamine, can lead to a psychosis in normal individuals; (ii) that positive symptoms of schizophrenic patients can be exacerbated by dopamine-releasing drugs; and (iii) all the clinically effective antipsychotic drugs in use today have the common property of blocking D_2 receptors (cf. Grace et al[1]). However, the concept that schizophrenia is due to a simple hyperdopaminergic state is not supported by a substantial amount of other evidence.

What is wrong with the dopamine hypothesis of schizophrenia? First, there is no evidence for the presence of abnormally high levels of dopamine or its metabolites in the brain of schizophrenic patients. We know that amphetamine, which is known to lead to schizophrenia in control subjects,[2] does so by causing a 30-fold elevation in extracellular dopamine in the brain, and certainly there is no evidence that there is any kind of increase of this magnitude in the brain of schizophrenic patients. Also, antipsychotic drugs can be administered at doses that can achieve any given level of receptor occupancy within minutes of their administration;[3] nonetheless, it takes weeks to get a maximal therapeutic action from these antipsychotic drugs.[4] In order to understand the therapeutic actions of the antipsychotic drugs, we need to know something about the limbic circuit and how dopamine influences this circuit. Basically, the prefrontal cortex provides a glutamatergic input to the nucleus accumbens which in turn activates a γ-aminobutyric

Nucleus accumbens circuits

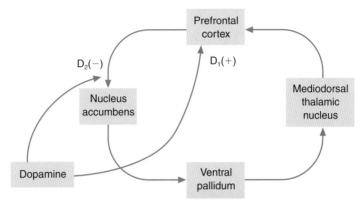

Figure 16.1 *Circuit diagram showing interactions of dopamine within the limbic circuit. The prefrontal cortex supplies a glutamatergic excitatory drive to the nucleus accumbens. The accumbens, in turn, provides a γ-aminobutyric acid (GABA)ergic inhibitory projection to the ventral pallidum, which itself provides a GABAergic inhibitory projection to the thalamus. Therefore, when the accumbens is activated, there is a disinhibition of the thalamus and excitation of the prefrontal cortex, completing this feedback facilitatory loop. Dopamine is capable of modulating this circuit at several points. In particular, a dopaminergic input from the ventral tegmental area facilitates activity within prefrontal cortical projection neurones via D_1 receptors. In contrast, dopamine at the level of the nucleus accumbens acts on D_2 receptors to attenuate prefrontal excitation of accumbens neurones via a presumed presynaptic inhibition of corticoaccumbens excitation. Antipsychotic drugs, which are primarily D_2 antagonists, would increase corticoaccumbens stimulation both by increasing dopamine release in the prefrontal cortex and by removing D_2-mediated inhibition of corticoaccumbens afferents.*

acid (GABA)ergic projection to the ventral pallidum and the mediodorsal thalamus. The thalamus provides an excitatory projection to the prefrontal cortex to complete this loop (Figure 16.1).

Dopamine has two important sites of action within this loop, at the level of the nucleus accumbens as well as within the prefrontal cortex. Of course because of the important role of dopamine in schizophrenia (see Figure 16.1), the effects of dopamine in these areas have been very well investigated. Yet trying to understand exactly what they do has been fraught with difficulty. Thus, when these systems have been examined in the intact organism in vivo, where there is not sufficient local pharmacological control over the neuronal environment, one can observe potent effects of dopaminergic drugs on neuronal activity. However, when examined in vitro, where there is better control over the access of drugs to the receptors at known concentrations, the effects are not as readily apparent.[5] This implies that a substantial portion of the effects of dopamine may depend on interactions between systems that are present in vivo but not in vitro. Therefore, we have approached this issue by employing a new technique in which the micro-dialysis probe is implanted, in this case for the purpose of administering drugs, and then in vivo intracellular recording in the area adjacent to the microdialysis probe is done, so that we can get a better idea of how changing the local environment affects the neuron recording front.[6]

Using this method in the prefrontal cortex, we tested the effects of dopamine on the activity of morphologically identified pyramidal neurones. At baseline, spontaneous low amplitude excitatory postsynaptic potentials (EPSPs) were observed. When N-methyl-D-aspartate (NMDA) was adminis-tered through the probe, an increase in the frequency of EPSPs and a depo-larization of the membrane were observed. Upon adding dopamine to the perfusate, we observed longer duration depolarization plateaus. Therefore, dopamine, acting via D_1 receptors, potentiated the response to glutamate within the prefrontal cortex. Subcortically within the nucleus accumbens, dopamine was also found to exert potent actions.[7] Specifically it has potent effects on the prefrontal cortical input to the accumbens. Using in vivo intracellular recording from accumbens neurones, it was found that adminis-tration of the D_2 antagonist eticlopride through the microdialysis probe caused an increase in the amplitude of EPSPs evoked by prefrontal cortical stimulation.[7] In contrast, administration of the D_1 antagonist did not cause this response. Since in this case a D_2 *antagonist* was found to increase the EPSP amplitude, this demonstrates that we are blocking a potent tonic inhi-bition of prefrontal cortical input exerted by endogenous levels of dopamine in the accumbens.

Overall, dopamine has divergent actions within this corticolimbic circuit, in which it activates the prefrontal cortex through D_1 receptors while inhibiting the prefrontal cortical stimulation of the nucleus accumbens via presynaptic D_2 receptors (see Figure 16.1). Current antipsychotic drugs are thought to be blocking the D_2 receptors in the accumbens and removing inhibition of corticoaccumbens fibres. Hopefully, with either D_1 agonists or potentially some glutamatergic modulatory drugs we can provide a means to activate this circuit to restore this cortical–subcortical balance in trying to maintain system function at normal levels.

Another variant that has a potent influence is the hippocampus, especially the hippocampus subiculum. It has been shown in a number of studies that this provides a powerful influence as far as focusing information flow within this circuit.[8] But recent data also show that the hippocampus itself has a rather potent effect on the dopamine innervation within the nucleus accumbens.[9] Specifically, when the ventral subiculum is activated by infusion of NMDA, the resultant activation of subicular multisynaptic efferent pathways to the ventral tegmental area causes an activation of dopamine neurones. Studies show that there are several indices of dopamine neurone population activity that can be used as a measure of the electro-physiological outflow from this region. Although dopamine neurones can change their firing rate, this is a rather limited parameter, given the con-straints on maximal firing rate of these neurones. But there are two other parameters that seem to be more important in regulating dopamine outflow: one is the overall activity of the dopamine neurones, in other words how many cells are actually firing, and the other is the firing pattern. It is known from the work of Schultz et al[10] and others that bursting activity within these cells seems to be more important in some of the behavioural indices of mea-surement within this system. We find that when NMDA is added there is very little change in either firing rate or burst firing of the dopamine neu-rones. On the other hand, there is a potent activation as far as the number of cells firing. Thus, NMDA infusion into the subiculum results in an activation of non-firing neurones. This seems to depend on this pathway acting via the accumbens, because infusion of the glutamate antagonist into the accumbens eliminates the effects of activating the hippocampus on dopamine neurone firing.

We then investigated the pathways from the accumbens to the ventral tegmental dopamine neurones that could mediate this activation. First, to mimic the activation of accumbens GABAergic output neurones by the ventral subiculum, GABAergic tone was increased within one of the primary targets of the accumbens: the ventral pallidum. This was done by infusing GABA A and GABA B agonists muscimol and baclofen into this region. When the ventral pallidum was inactivated by this infusion, there again was no change in dopamine neurone firing rate or pattern, but there was a sub-stantial increase in the number of dopamine cells firing. So our view is that the ventral pallidum, because of its high rate of firing, is holding subsets of cells in the ventral tegmental area inhibited, while allowing the other cells to fire. When we inactivated the ventral pallidum, this inhibition was relieved, allowing more dopamine neurones to initiate spontaneous spike firing.

Another pathway that is likely to be affected via the accumbens output system is the pedunculopontine nucleus. This system is known to provide glutamatergic and cholinergic innervation to the ventral tegmental area. In this case we activated this input by infusion of the GABAergic antagonist bicuculline. There was no change in firing rate, nor was there a change in population activity, but what we did find was a very powerful increase in burst firing.

Therefore, by manipulating these pathways we can independently regulate the number of dopamine cells firing versus burst firing. This enabled us to examine the relative impact of these two parameters of dopamine cell activity and how it affects dopamine release in the accumbens. This was done by implanting a microdialysis probe within the accumbens and manipulating these systems. First, inactivation of the ventral pallidum, which would increase the number of dopamine neurones firing, led to a 50% increase in extracellular dopamine levels in the accumbens. Therefore, activation of silent, non-firing dopamine neurones leads to increased dopamine levels. What about the effect of increasing burst firing? This is something that we would predict to have potent effects on dopamine release, because this type of activity is most often associated with behaviourally relevant stimuli. However, activation of the pedunculopontine caused no change in extracellular dopamine levels. This is surprising, because we know that activating the pedunculopontine will activate dopamine-mediated behaviours that can be blocked with dopamine antagonists. In order to investigate this, we gave the drug nomifensine through the dialysis probe. Nomifensine blocks dopamine uptake. Whenever dopamine uptake is blocked, a nine-fold increase in extracellular dopamine can initially be measured. Nonetheless, despite this large increase in baseline, inactivation of the ventral pallidum yields approximately the same 50% increase in extracellular dopamine levels. So although there are of course much higher levels of dopamine being released given the higher baseline, the proportional increase is the same as in the absence of nomifensine administration.

What happens whenever burst firing is caused by activating the pedunculopontine nucleus? Despite the nine-fold increase in baseline dopamine, activation of the pedunculopontine causes a 300% increase over this elevated baseline with respect to extracellular dopamine levels, but only in the presence of the reuptake blocker nomifensine. This suggests that there is a markedly different dynamic regulation of dopamine by these two afferent systems. Changes in the number of cells firing causes a proportionate change in the extracellular dopamine levels that is not impacted by the reuptake system. On the other hand, burst firing appears to cause a marked increase in dopamine release; however, this is not apparent unless reuptake is first blocked. We think that this can be explained on the basis of what can be called the tonic–phasic model of dopamine system dynamics.[11] In other words, burst firing causes a very large increase in dopamine release. This burst firing is activated by behaviourally salient stimuli as described by Wolfram Schultz[10] and others that have recorded from dopamine neurones in behaving animals. But this enormous increase in synaptic dopamine is immediately removed by the dopamine reuptake process without escaping the synaptic cleft, and therefore is not measurable as a change in extracellular dopamine levels. In contrast, the slow single-spike firing which we know is necessary to measure extrasynaptic dopamine, is the main drive of this tonic extracellular dopamine level that we can measure with dialysis. This is dependent on dopamine cell firing, and is likely to be modulated by presynaptic glutamatergic actions in the accumbens.[11] Although the tonic dopamine levels are less than 1/1000th of the intrasynaptic dopamine level, these extracellular concentrations are still capable of stimulating presynaptic dopamine autoreceptors, thereby decreasing phasic dopamine release. Therefore, I had proposed that this balance between cortically modulated tonic dopamine levels and burst firing-mediated phasic dopamine release is essential for understanding the dynamics of dopamine system regulation.

In order to assess what impact this system may have with respect to psychiatric disorders, we attempted to develop an animal model of schizophrenia. Of course, mimicking a complex cognitive disturbance such as schizophrenia in a rat is fraught with confounds; however, we attempted to achieve this by taking advantage of evidence that disruption during development is likely to play a role in the pathophysiology of schizophrenia in humans. To do this the drug methylazoxymethanol acetate (MAM) was used. This drug is known to interfere with DNA replication and neuronal development. It was given to pregnant rats during gestational day 17, which is the time when some of the limbic cortical areas are developing. To briefly summarize our results on this model, we find that it has a lot of anatomical correspondence with schizophrenia.[12] There is a thinning of limbic cortical structures that occurs with an increase of cell packing density, similarly to what has been reported in schizophrenic patients. With behavioural evidence we see disruption of pre-pulse inhibition of startle and impairment in reversal learning indicative of perseveration. Pharmacologically, these animals show increased responses to phencyclidine (PCP), as well as increased locomotion to amphetamine in the adult but not in the prepubertal animal. Therefore, this model exhibits many features consistent with what one would predict for an animal model of this disorder. When the dopamine system of MAM-treated rats as adults was examined, it was found that the dopamine neurones show more burst firing, and that ketamine has a stronger effect on decreasing spontaneous firing rate. But we observe a reversing of the effects of ketamine on burst firing, whereby it goes from an inhibition to an excitation. What we are doing in the case of these MAM-treated animals is increasing dopamine system function as far as burst firing is concerned, but decreasing the tonic levels. In other words, this tonic–phasic dopamine balance is being disturbed. We are decreasing the brake on the system by decreasing the spontaneous slow firing which contributes to the extracellular tonic dopamine levels, while exacerbating burst firing-mediated synaptic dopamine release. This could explain why this dysregulation that is occurring with cortical regulation of subcortical dopamine systems results in too much dopamine function as evidenced by studies such as those of Marc Laruelle, in which amphetamine administration causes significantly higher dopamine release in schizophrenic patients compared with controls, even though the basal state of the dopamine system appears normal.[13] Therefore, our evidence supports a model of schizophrenia in which cortical regulation of subcortical dopamine systems is disrupted, with the aetiology derived from an early developmental insult to these cortical systems.[14]

References

1. Grace AA, Bunney BS, Moore H, Todd CL, Dopamine cell depolarization block as a model for the therapeutic actions of antipsychotic drugs. *Trends Neurosci* 1997; 20:31–37.
2. Angrist B, Santhananthan G, Wilk S, Gershon S, Amphetamine psychosis: behavioral and biochemical aspects. *J Psychiatr Res* 1974; 11:13–23.
3. Sedvall G, Farde L, Persson A, Wiesel F-A, Imaging of neurotransmitter receptors in the living human brain. *Arch Gen Psychiatry* 1986; 43:995–1005.
4. Johnstone EC, Crow TJ, Frith CD, Carney MWP, Price JS, Mechanism of the antipsychotic effect in the treatment of acute schizophrenia. *Lancet* 1978; 22:848–851.
5. Grace AA, Dopamine. In: Charney D, Coyle J, Davis K, Nemeroff C (eds), *Psychopharmacology: The Fifth Generation of Progress*. Lippincott, Williams and Wilkins, Raven Press: New York, 2002.
6. West AR, Moore H, Grace AA, Direct examination of local regulation of membrane activity in striatal and prefrontal cortical neurons in vivo using simultaneous intracellular recording and microdialysis. *J Pharmacol Exp Ther* 2002; 301:867–877.
7. West AR, Grace AA, Opposite influences of endogenous dopamine D1 and D2 receptor activation on activity states and electrophysiological properties of striatal

neurons: studies combining in vivo intracellular recordings and reverse micro-dialysis. *J Neurosci* 2002; **22**:294–304.

8. O'Donnell P, Grace AA, Synaptic interactions among excitatory afferents to nucleus accumbens neurons: hippocampal gating of prefrontal cortical input. *J Neurosci* 1995; **15**:3622–3639.

9. Floresco SB, West AR, Ash B, Moore H, Grace AA, Ventral pallidal and pedunculo-pontine regulation of mesolimbic dopamine neuron activity: electrophysiological and neurochemical analyses. *Soc Neurosci Abstr* 2002; **28**:Program No. 358.4.

10. Schultz W, Tremblay L, Hollerman JR, Reward prediction in primate basal ganglia and frontal cortex. *Neuropharmacology* 1998; **37**:421–429.

11. Grace AA, Phasic versus tonic dopamine release and the modulation of dopamine system responsivity: a hypothesis for the etiology of schizophrenia. *Neuroscience* 1991; **41**:1–24.

12. Grace AA, Moore H, Regulation of information flow in the nucleus accumbens: a model for the pathophysiology of schizophrenia. In: Lenzenweger MF, Dworkin RH (eds) *Origins and Development of Schizophrenia: Advances in experimental psychopathology*. American Psychological Association Press: Washington, DC, 1998.

13. Laruelle M, Abi-Dargham A, Dopamine as the wind of the psychotic fire: new evidence from brain imaging studies. *J Psychopharmacol* 1999; **13**:358–371.

14. Grace AA, Developmental dysregulation of the dopamine system and the pathophysiology of schizophrenia. In: Keshavan M, Kennedy JL, Murray RM (eds), *Neurodevelopment and Schizophrenia*. Cambridge University Press, Cambridge, 2003.

chapter 17

Schizophrenia is a disorder of consciousness

Chris Frith

In contrast to many other contributors the title of this chapter was chosen by me (rather than being provided by the editors). I chose it to challenge all those people who are trying to develop animal models of schizophrenia. The kind of symptoms that interest me in particular – the delusions and the hallucinations – cannot be studied directly in mice or rats. They are disorders of consciousness[1] that are only known about from the subjective reports of patients. This chapter focuses on the kinds of delusions where patients believe they are being controlled by external forces in some way. Interestingly, two big studies showed that the severity of delusions and hallucinations is not associated with impairments on typical neuropsychological tests.[2,3] This observation suggests that the cognitive deficits associated with hallucinations and delusions are not tapped by standard tests of cognitive function.

Another kind of orthodoxy that I would like to challenge in this chapter concerns Karl Jaspers' idea that these problems in schizophrenia are simply not understandable.[4] I will try to show that we can understand them: at the level of psychology, physiology and in experiential terms to get some idea of what it is like to have these symptoms, and that there is in fact a link between the mind and the brain. Everyone plays lip service to this idea, but in my view, other than this chapter, only Chapter 14 addresses this point in this book. In the rest of the book the emphasis is in on either the brain or the mind and not on the link between the two. The nearest that most schizophrenia researchers have come to making such a link is, for example, 'hallucinations are caused by supersensitive dopamine receptors'. There is clearly an explanatory gap here which this chapter aims to try to fill. This, of course, is the programme of cognitive neuroscience. It is cognitive models which can make the link between neural activity in the brain on the one hand and behaviour and subjective experience on the other.

The 'anarchic hand' versus delusions of control

The most famous example of an anarchic hand was experienced by one of Peter Seller's many characters in the film *Dr Strangelove*. The interesting feature of this particular case was that the hand in question was an artificial one. In reality, the anarchic hand is an extremely interesting but rather rare neurological disorder where one hand moves of its own accord without the patient wanting it to. It grasps door knobs, picks up and uses pencils and so on.[5] What is interesting is what the patients think about this behaviour. They recognize that the hand's movements are unintended. In one case, for example, the patient tried to prevent the hand from moving by holding it with her other hand or tying it to the bed overnight. These patients do not believe that they are being controlled by alien forces. They believe that there is something wrong with their hand. This is a striking contrast with delusions of control, where patients feel that their actions are controlled by alien forces. In Sean Spence's classic experiment on delusions of control (see below) the patients were performing a fairly simple task, in which they had to move a joystick in a sequence of random directions. They did this task correctly, but they still reported that they were being controlled by alien forces. In this case the hand was doing what they intended it to do, because they were successfully performing the task and yet they experienced the hand as being controlled by some outside force. This is not a disorder of motor control as is the case with the anarchic hand. This is a disorder of the *awareness* of motor control. In particular, I want to suggest that the problem lies in an excessive awareness of the sensory consequences of action. However, first we must consider awareness in the normal motor system.

Normal awareness of motor control

How much are we normally aware of our own movements and of the systems that control these movements? In one of the first studies to address this issue Benjamin Libet (Libet et al[6]) asked people to do a very simple task: they had to lift one finger whenever they felt like it. This act is associated in the electroencephalogram (EEG) with a potential, which becomes slowly more negative for about 1 sec before the finger is actually moved. Libet's ingenious idea was to ask people to indicate two things. First, at what time they had the urge to move their finger, and second, at what time they actually lifted their finger. The most interesting observation in my view was that the time at which they thought they lifted their finger was reliably about 80 msec before the finger was actually lifted. This result has been replicated.[7] So what are you aware of if you are aware of lifting your finger about 80 msec before the finger is actually moved? It cannot be awareness of the sensory feedback resulting from the lifting, because this will not be available until 100 msec or so after the finger has been lifted. Presumably, what you are aware of is not the actual consequences of lifting your finger, but the expected consequences of lifting the finger. These consequences can be predicted on the basis of the muscle commands that were initiated to make the finger move.

There is another interesting feature of the Libet result that has been extensively discussed. The time at which people report having the urge to lift their finger is about 300 msec after detectable changes in EEG activity. Although some people think this observation eliminates the possibility of free will, it is interesting that in the mental domain the urge to lift the finger and the actual moment of lifting it are closer together in time than in the physical domain. In the mental domain the urge to lift is experienced as later and the moment of lifting is experienced as earlier. This is a form of binding that Patrick Haggard calls 'intentional binding' between the intention to lift and the actual lift.[7] This effect enhances one's sense of agency, the feeling of being in control of one's actions. Patrick Haggard has shown that the same binding effect is achieved when studying the lifting of a finger and some event caused by it, e.g. hearing a buzzer. Here again the times of these two events in the mental domain are pulled together, thus increasing the experience of causing the buzzer to sound by lifting the finger. When the experience of causality is disrupted by using transcranial magnetic stimulation (TMS) to cause the movement, then the times of the two events are pulled apart in the mental domain.[8]

There are two things that are important in these observations. First, the awareness is not of the actual sensory feedback from moving the finger, but some prediction about the sensation (see also Fourneret and Jeannerod[9] for an example of lack of awareness of sensory feedback). Second, in the mental domain the causes and effects are pulled together in time. This may have the effect of enhancing the sense of being in control of one's own actions.

Daniel Wolpert has developed a model of motor control which explains how the prediction of the sensory consequences might be achieved (see for example Frith et al[10]). If the goal is to reach out with the hand and press a button, then the first thing to do is work out the sequence of motor commands that will achieve this goal. This computation is called 'inverse modelling' and depends upon a controller. On the basis of this computation and before any movements are made, one can compute what would happen if these motor commands were issued and also what sensations would occur. This is called 'forward modelling' and depends upon a predictor. Such a system predicts in advance what sensations will occur when any act is carried out. The predicted sensations can be compared with the actual sensations that follow. If they do not match, then something unexpected has happened. What one is aware of when a movement is made is the *predicted* sensation. Awareness of the actual sensations is there only if there is a big discrepancy from those predicted. There is no need to experience sensations already known about because they have been successfully predicted.

This, of course, is the reason why you can't tickle yourself. When you tickle yourself, you can predict in advance what you're going to feel, and therefore the feeling is attenuated. An elegant experiment by Sarah-Jayne Blakemore demonstrated the precision of this prediction (Blakemore et al[11]). She used two robot arms. The first robot arm recorded the movements the volunteer made with their right hand and transferred these movements to the second robot arm that reproduced them on the volunteer's left hand. This made the volunteer feel as if they were tickling themselves with a rigid metal rod and did not feel very ticklish. If the robot tickled the volunteer all by itself, using the movements previously recorded, it felt much more ticklish. Using this system, time delays, of say 200 msec, were introduced between the volunteer's and the robot's movements; as the delay increased, the ticklishness also increased showing that the awareness of the sensation depended precisely on the prediction. Interestingly, at the 200-msec delay it was as ticklish as if the robot was making the movements by itself, even though the volunteer was not aware of the delay.

These effects can also be seen in the physiological domain. In another study volunteers were having magnetic resonance imaging (MRI) scans while being tickled using a special wooden tickling device that works inside strong magnetic fields.[12] The secondary somatosensory cortex (SII) was activated bilaterally when the volunteers were tickled. This region was activated much less when the volunteers were tickling themselves and indeed it was not activated any more than if they were simply moving their right hand, but not actually tickling themselves. So this activity was almost entirely attenuated when it was self-produced.

Do patients with delusions of control lack attenuation of self-generated sensations?

The critical prediction is that patients with delusions of control and related passivity disorders should not show the normal attenuation of sensations associated with self-produced movements. In other words, they should be able to tickle themselves. This was studied by Sarah-Jayne Blakemore in collaboration with Eve Johnstone's group in Edinburgh. Three groups of patients, those with passivity symptoms, those with other psychotic symptoms and also control subjects were tested. The control subjects and the patients not having passivity experiences showed the normal pattern, that is that there is less subjective sensation when you are tickling yourself, and more effect when someone else is tickling you. In the patients with delusions of control and related symptoms, there was no difference in reported sensation between tickling themselves and somebody else tickling them. This result suggests that there is something wrong with the attenuation system concerned with self-produced actions in patients with these particular symptoms.

There is indirect evidence for similar lack of attenuation in the physiological domain. Sean Spence and colleagues carried out a very elegant experiment using positron emission tomography (PET).[14] Patients who were currently suffering from delusions of control carried out a simple motor task. In many cases they actually experienced delusions of control while they were being scanned. They were compared with patients without the delusions and control subjects. Patients with delusions of control showed overactivity in the right parietal cortex. Furthermore, this overactivity disappeared when the patients were tested some months later when the symptoms were no longer present. Thus the overactivity seemed to be specifically related to the presence of delusions of control.

It is my belief that this overactivity reflects a lack of attenuation of the activity associated with sensations associated with the hand and arm movements associated with the motor task. Cornelius Weiller and colleagues contrasted activity associated with active and passive arm movements in normal volunteers.[15] This was not tickling but a comparison of the volunteer moving their hand or someone else moving their hand. During passive movements, there was greater activity in a region of the parietal cortex close to SII. Again, during self-generated movements activity in the parietal cortex was attenuated.

This result suggests that, when schizophrenic patients with delusions of control move their hands, they show a pattern of brain activity that looks like normal people having their hands passively moved. I would argue that for them it really does feel as if their arms were being moved by external forces.

We recently carried out an experiment in collaboration with David Oakley in which hypnosis was used to create an experience of alien control in normal volunteers.[16] Under hypnosis it is standard practice to tell subjects that their arms will move up and down all by themselves. The subject will then actively make arm movements that are experienced as passive. During such movements there is greater activity in the parietal cortex than during identical active movements that are experienced as active.

This mechanism of attenuation not only allows one to ignore irrelevant sensory events because they are caused by oneself and are not interesting, but also is critical for the experience of agency, i.e. the experience of being in control of self-produced actions. Farrer and Frith examined this problem directly by asking volunteers to decide whether they or someone else was controlling the movements of a pointer on a computer screen.[17] When the movement is actually caused by somebody else, again more activity is seen in the parietal cortex. There are now several experiments suggesting that in normal controls this region is particularly involved in distinguishing actions caused by other people and actions caused by the self.[18]

These experiments suggest that lack of attenuation of activity in the parietal cortex is associated, not only with the experience that one is not actively moving, but also with the experience that someone else is moving. This observation provides a plausible account of the proximal origin of the experience of delusions of control. Note that I am not implying that this area of the parietal cortex must be abnormal in schizophrenia but that over-activity in this area seems to relate to some of the symptoms of schizophrenia. It may well be that the lack of attenuation results from the failure of top-down control from some other region of the brain, most likely the pre-frontal cortex. This hypothesis can be explored further be examining the relation between measures of functional connectivity and the presence of symptoms (e.g. Lawrie et al[19]).

Conclusion

What might it be like to have delusions of control? Although the situation in the following example hardly exists anymore today because of the widespread use of computerized presentations, in the good old days when people used carousel projectors there were many ways in which things could go wrong. Some projectors would advance slides at random moments or because of noises in the street. This is an example of an 'anarchic' projector and the obvious conclusion would be that there was something wrong with the projector. But there is another, very different scenario in which the projector behaves in an unexpected way. Consider a meeting where you are speaking after a lecturer who never mastered the control of visual aids. He tapped on the floor with his long wooden pointer to indicate that the next slide should be shown. You, of course, are prepared to advance your own slides by pressing the button on the lectern. But just as you reach to press the button, the slide advances all by itself. This is a delusion of alien control for a carousel projector. You intended to advance the projector, but some alien force advanced it for you. You might believe that there must be some agent controlling the projector who can read your mind, and in this case you would be right. It is the projectionist in her box who can predict from the talk when you want to change the slide. In conclusion, this is what I think a delusion of alien control might feel like.

References

1. Frith CD, Consciousness, information processing and schizophrenia. *Bri J Psychiatry* 1979; **134**:225–235.
2. Johnstone EC, Frith CD, Validation of three dimensions of schizophrenic symptoms in a large unselected sample of patients. *Psychol Med* 1996; **26**:669–679.
3. Basso MR, Nasrallah HA, Olson SC, Bornstein RA, Neuropsychological correlates of negative, disorganized and psychotic symptoms in schizophrenia. *Schizophr Res* 1998; **31**:99–111.
4. Jaspers K, *General Psychopathology*. Manchester University Press: Manchester, 1962.
5. Marchetti C, Della Salla S, Disentangling the alien and anarchic hand. *Cogn Neuropsychiatry* 1998; **3**:191–208.
6. Libet B, Gleason CA, Wright EW, Pearl DK, Time of conscious intention to act in relation to onset of cerebral activity (readiness-potential). The unconscious initiation of a freely voluntary act. *Brain* 1983; **106**:623–642.
7. Haggard P, Newman C, Magno E, On the perceived time of voluntary actions. *Br J Psychology* 1999; **90**:291–303.
8. Haggard P, Clark S, Kalogeras J, Voluntary action and conscious awareness. *Nat Neurosci* **5**:382–385.
9. Fourneret P, Jeannerod M, Limited conscious monitoring of motor performance in normal subjects. *Neuropsychologia* 1998; **36**:1133–1140.

10. Frith CD, Blakemore SJ, Wolpert DM, Abnormalities in the awareness and control of action. *Philos Trans R Soc Lon* 2000; **355**:1771–1788.

11. Blakemore SJ, Frith CD, Wolpert DM, Spatio-temporal prediction modulates the perception of self-produced stimuli. *J Cogn Neurosci* 1999; **11**:551–559.

12. Blakemore SJ, Wolpert DM, Frith CD, Central cancellation of self-produced tickle sensation. *Nat Neurosci* 1998; **1**:635–640.

13. Blakemore S-J, Smith J, Steel RM, Johnstone EC, Frith CD, The perception of self-produced sensory stimuli in patients with auditory hallucinations and passivity experiences: evidence for a breakdown in self-monitoring. *Psychol Med* 2000; **30**:1131–1139.

14. Spence SA, Brooks DJ, Hirsch SR, Liddle PF, Meehan J, Grasby PM, A PET study of voluntary movement in schizophrenic patients experiencing passivity phenomena (delusions of alien control). *Brain* 1997; **120**:1997–2011.

15. Weiller C, Juptner M, Fellows S et al, Brain representation of active and passive movements. *Neuroimage* 1996; **4**:105–110.

16. Blakemore SJ, Oakley DA, Frith CD, Delusions of alien control in the normal brain. *Neuropsychologia* 2003; **41**:1058–1067.

17. Farrer C, Frith CD, Experiencing oneself vs another person as being the cause of an action: the neural correlates of the experience of agency. *Neuroimage* 2001; **15**:596–603.

18. Meltzoff AN, Decety J, What imitation tells us about social cognition: a rapprochement between developmental psychology and cognitive neuroscience. *Philos Trans R Soc Lond B Biol Sci* **358**:491–500.

19. Lawrie SM, Buechel C, Whalley HC, Frith CD, Friston KJ, Johnstone EC, Reduced frontotemporal functional connectivity in schizophrenia associated with auditory hallucinations. *Biol Psychiatry* 2002; **51**:1008–1011.

chapter 18

Does cognitive behaviour therapy work in schizophrenia?

Shôn Lewis

The notion that the core symptoms of schizophrenia might be amenable to psychological treatments until recently bordered on the heretical. Schizophrenia was a biological disorder and there was accepted evidence that not only was interpretative psychotherapy useless, it might actively be harmful.[1]

Over the past 10 years, there has been increasing interest, particularly in the UK and Europe, in the possibility that specific and specifiable psychological treatments can be effective in reducing the symptoms of schizophrenia. The widest claims have been made for cognitive behaviour therapy (CBT). What is the evidence for this?

The evidence

The evidence base for psychological treatments in schizophrenia is summarized in Box 18.1, which lists those interventions supported by at least one good quality clinical trial.

Box 18.1 Effective psychological interventions in schizophrenia

- Psychoeducation
- Family interventions[2]
- Motivational interviewing for comorbid substance use[3]
- Compliance therapy for medication non-adherence[4]
- Cognitive behaviour therapy
- Cognitive remediation for neurocognitive deficits[5]

The effectiveness of CBT is now supported by a sizeable body of evidence, although the first trials in this area were undertaken in the mid-1990s. The best replicated findings are that CBT, if delivered over a sustained period, will reduce positive and to some extent negative symptoms in otherwise treatment-resistant schizophrenia. In these trials, as with all others so far, CBT has been delivered as an adjunct to drug treatment as usual. Four independent, high quality, trials[6-9] used similar inclusion criteria, patients with persistent symptoms despite adequate treatment with two or more antipsychotic drugs, with similar experimental treatments in terms of content and duration – 6–9 months. The trials differed in other respects, particularly the selection of control interventions and the use or otherwise of blinded assessments of outcome. Overall, the effect size for improvement of positive symptoms in these trials is about 0.6. Some improvement was also seen in negative symptoms and, in some circumstances, social functioning. In addition, the effect appears to be durable at 6–9 months post-treatment and beyond. In the trial of Sensky et al,[7] the effect of the control intervention, befriending, appeared not to extend beyond the end of treatment, whereas the effect of CBT seemed actually to consolidate over the follow-up period. Box 18.2 lists the aspects of schizophrenia for which the effectiveness of CBT has been demonstrated.

The patient population in these trials is similar to that of the earlier clozapine efficacy studies and the effect size, according to a systematic review, is about the same.[10] An important statistical issue here is that the population and the samples drawn from for these trials are selected on the basis of having persistent and stable positive symptoms, so maximizing the power of a trial to

---

Box 18.2 Aspects of schizophrenia where cognitive behaviour therapy has been shown to be effective: quality of evidence from randomized control trials

• Persistent positive symptoms	+++
• Negative symptoms	++
• Acute episode	+
• First episode	++
• Relapse prevention	++
• 'Prodromal' symptoms	++

+: one trial of equivocal design; ++: one trial of good design; +++: 2 or more trials

test the efficacy of an add-on treatment. This statistical advantage may not be present when other patient populations are targeted, such as first episode or acutely ill patients, or patients in remission open to relapse.

The results of these trials have been taken up enthusiastically by a clinical community looking for alternative strategies to drug treatments. Patients also have welcomed this new line of evidence. It is not surprising that people suffering from, or caring for, those with severe psychological symptoms should expect treatments based on primary psychological approaches to be available. It is important to recognize that some of the more recent trials suffer from methodological limitations, particularly those which could lead to a type 1 statistical error, where a false positive result is found.

The design features of a good clinical trial are shown in Box 18.3. In general, it can be argued that the ground rules for establishing the effectiveness of psychological treatments should be no different from those used to establish effectiveness of pharmacological treatments. Moreover, it can be argued that the closer the design specifications and the choice of clinical outcomes between drug and non-drug trials, the more statements can be made comparing the two approaches.

Looking at specific issues, the use of a double blind design, as is the benchmark approach in phase III clinical trials of a drug treatment, is not possible with psychological treatments. This makes it more, rather than less, important that where blindness of outcome assessment is possible, it is used. There have been debates about whether or not it is possible to maintain a blind to treatment allocation when assessing outcome. Because of the known potency of the use of non-blind assessments in introducing bias, is vital to attempt to use independent, blind assessments of outcome, with assessment of the quality of the blind if possible. In addition, the choice of outcomes

---

Box 18.3 Design features of a good psychological treatment trial

- Large, representative sample from clinically relevant population
- Sample size justified by power calculation
- Independent randomization
- Well specified intervention whose fidelity is independently assessed
- Outcomes assessed blind to treatment allocation
- Reliable and valid primary outcome measure
- Intent to treat analysis with description of dropouts

should include those which are relatively impermeable to the effects of blindness, such as relapse, hospitalization and instrumental outcomes such as employment status.

There has been a trend of late to focus on pragmatic trials in health care generally. These are trials which tend to be large with simple outcomes which solely address the question of effectiveness. It can be argued that in an area such as psychological treatments of psychosis it is vital to build into trial design an explanatory component to test whether the hypothesized mechanism is actually that which mediates any effect. One example would be that the clinical effect of a psychological treatment is actually mediated inadvertently through another therapeutic mechanism, such as improved adherence to drug treatments. Another important issue specific to this area is replicability. With CBT, this typically involves a range of individual psychological techniques. It is important that the objective demonstration of treatment fidelity, that is that the treatment given adheres to a written procedural protocol, is measured and reported.

How might cognitive behaviour therapy work?

In general, the aetiological model in schizophrenia which underlies this area is the stress-vulnerability model. In this model, an underlying biological vulnerability to schizophrenia is necessary but not sufficient to produce the final phenotype. Because psychological treatments might be effective in reducing the symptoms of schizophrenia does not negate the importance of biological mechanisms, in the same way that the efficacy of drug treatments might negate the possible importance of psychological factors.

Cognitive models of how positive psychotic symptoms might arise have become well developed. The model outlined by Garety and colleagues[11] outlines the steps which might be involved and has some empirical basis. The first step is the generation of anomalous conscious experiences. The model supposes that some individuals are prone to such experiences as a result of a longstanding information processing trait. One such trait is that proposed by Hemsley,[12] where a weakened influence of stored memories of regularities of previous input gives rise to the experience of unfamiliarity to everyday perceptions. Another trait is that put forward by Frith,[13] where a deficit in the normal, automatic process of self-monitoring of intentions and actions results in the misattribution of internally generated events to the external world. Either mechanism (Figure 18.1) might play a part in producing the

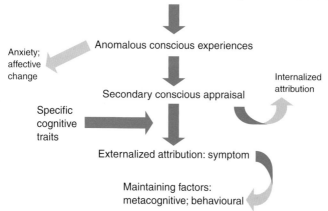

Intrusion of stored memories[13] or deficit in self-monitoring of intentions and actions[14]

Figure 18.1 Cognitive mechanisms in symptom formation.

type of anomalous experience which recent epidemiological work has suggested is relatively frequent in the general community, appearing as non-syndromal, isolated hallucinatory phenomena, for example.

Next in the chain of events is the conscious appraisal by the individual of the nature of these anomalous phenomena. Usually, the phenomena will be rejected as abnormal and put down to factors such as stress, intoxication or fatigue. In some people, however, the presence of a further set of cognitive traits will not allow this rejection. These traits might include the presence of an externalizing attributional style, or deficits in social cognition, such as theory of mind, or a particular style of information gathering, which reaches judgements on the basis of inadequate data, a style of 'jumping to conclusions'. The result is that, rather than being attributed correctly to internal events, the unusual phenomena begin to be attributed mistakenly to external agencies. This process may be made more likely, or accelerated, if the phenomena produce or occur in the context of states of distress or anxiety. The final stages involve consolidation and then maintenance of the newly formed psychotic phenomena, again involving a further set of cognitive traits, such as metacognitive appraisals of controllability and the adoption of safety behaviours which serve to maintain the symptoms.

Whether CBT acts on core psychotic symptoms to produce improved outcome can be debated. In related areas of psychological treatment in schizophrenia, it is explicit that the psychological treatment is operating to enhance the effect of a known, external protective factor, or to reduce the effect of a known risk factor. An example of the former is the psychological intervention in so-called compliance therapy where the psychological treatment is aimed at enhancing the known protective effect of taking pre-scribed antipsychotic drug treatments.[4,14] An example of reducing a specific risk factor is the trial of motivational and family interventions in patients with schizophrenia and comorbid street drug use, where the focus of psycho-logical treatment was the established link between street drug use and relapse.[3]

In some trials, the effects of CBT are intended to be mediated at least in part through the moderation of risk and protective factors, except this time these are not external, but secondary aspects of psychopathology. The best example of this is the model of CBT based on coping-strategy enhancement[6] in which the psychological treatment specifically accesses and aims to enhance strategies already developed by the individual to cope with con-tinuing psychotic symptoms. Another example would be the use of psycho-logical strategies to reduce anxiety and depression which usually exist alongside primary psychotic symptoms and serve to maintain them. Again, the use of measures to assess independently these aspects of psy-chopathology in trials is important in trying to understand how these psy-chological techniques exert their effect.

In addition to persistent symptoms, there is some evidence that CBT can accelerate resolution of symptoms in the acute episode.[15] To evaluate effec-tiveness in the acute symptoms in early schizophrenia, Lewis et al[16] con-ducted a large trial of 315 cases of first and second admissions for schizophrenia randomized to one of three treatment conditions: routine care alone, or routine care plus supportive counselling as a control for non-specific effects, or routine care plus a 5-week package of CBT. Short-term out-comes showed that adding CBT accelerated average time to remission, from about 6 weeks to 4 weeks. Eighteen-month follow-up showed that sympto-matic outcomes were slightly but significantly better in the CBT group, but there was no effect on time to relapse. One high quality trial has shown CBT to be effective in postponing relapse in patients selected to be 'relapse prone' on the basis of their recent history.[17] Predictors of good treatment response are listed in Box 18.4.

Box 18.4 Predictors of good treatment response to cognitive behaviour therapy (CBT)

- Number of treatment sessions; treatment duration
- Good therapeutic alliance
- Younger age
- Partial insight
- Auditory hallucinations
- Emphasis on behavioural aspects of CBT

Can cognitive behaviour therapy prevent schizophrenia?

Very early intervention in psychotic disorders has recently become a focus of research. A small number of studies have examined the possibility of detecting individuals in the prodromal stage, prior to the development of full psychosis. Yung and colleagues[18] pioneered this approach to prevention, with operational criteria to identify four subgroups at ultra-high risk of incipient psychosis. In their initial sample, 40% made the transition to psychosis over a 9-month period. The improved ability accurately to define high risk has led to the prospect of primary, or at least early secondary, prevention.

McGorry and colleagues[19] showed that pharmacotherapy with low dose risperidone, plus CBT, reduced the rate of transition to psychosis in young people at ultra-high risk, in comparison with supportive therapy and case management. This protective effect did not persist at follow-up, after discontinuation of drug treatment and CBT. The relative contributions of drug treatment and psychotherapy could not be determined since this was a combined treatment.

Morrison et al[20] hypothesized that CBT alone would significantly reduce the transition rate in help seeking individuals meeting the same criteria, in comparison with the treatment as usual group. In a controlled trial, out of 58 participants who met criteria for being high risk according to the Yung et al[18] criteria, 33 were randomly allocated to CBT and 25 to a monitoring control. No participants had received antipsychotic medication at baseline. Participants were assessed for suitability and monitored on a monthly basis using the Positive and Negative Syndromes Scale (PANSS),[21] which was also used to determine transition. Of the 58 participants, 47 were recruited on the basis of attenuated psychotic symptoms.

An interim analysis included all patients, but only 38 had been followed up for the full 12 months (the rest had all been followed up for at least 6 months). Rates of PANSS-defined transition were as follows: two of 33 patients (6%) allocated to cognitive therapy made transition and four of 25 patients (16%) allocated to monitoring made transition. Predictor variables contributing to transition were shown to be initial PANSS positive score (B = 0.48; $P = 0.06$), age (B = 0.21; $P = 0.05$) and treatment group (B = 0.32; $P = 0.06$). These results suggest that cognitive therapy may be effective, during the active treatment phase, in reducing transition to psychosis in a high-risk group. This is the first study to suggest that CBT alone may prevent or delay progression to psychosis in the absence of drug treatment. This new treatment paradigm may clarify the cognitive mechanisms underlying the pathogenesis of psychotic symptoms.

References

1. Mueser KT, Berenbaum H, Psychodynamic treatment of schizophrenia: is there a future? *Psychol Med* 1990; **20**:253–62.
2. Pharoah FM, Mari JJ, Streiner D, Family intervention for schizophrenia. *Cochrane Database Syst Rev* 2000; **2**:CD000088.
3. Barrowclough C, Haddock G, Tarrier N et al, Randomized controlled trial of motivational interviewing, cognitive behavior therapy, and family intervention for patients with comorbid schizophrenia and substance use disorders. *Am J Psychiatry* 2001; **158**:1706–1713.
4. Kemp R, Hayward P, Applethwaite G, Everritt B, David A, Compliance therapy in psychotic patients: randomised controlled trial. *BMJ* 1996; **312**:345–349.
5. Wykes T, Reeder C, Corner J, Williams C, Everitt B, The effects of neurocognitive remediation on executive processing in patients with schizophrenia. *Schizophr Bull* 1999; **25**:291–307.
6. Tarrier N, Sharpe L, Beckett R, Harwood S, Baker A, Yusopoff L, A trial of two cognitive behavioural methods of treating drug-resistant residual psychotic symptoms in schizophrenic patients. II. Treatment-specific changes in coping and problem-solving skills. *Soc Psychiatry Psychiatr Epidemiol* 1993; **28**:5–10.
7. Sensky T, Turkington T, Kingdon D et al, A randomised, controlled trial of cognitive behaviour therapy for persistent positive symptoms in schizophrenia resistant to medication. *Arch Gen Psychiatry* 2000; **57**:165–173.
8. Tarrier N, Yusopoff L, Kinney C et al, Randomised controlled trial of intensive cognitive behaviour therapy for patients with chronic schizophrenia. *BMJ* 1998; **317**:303–307.
9. Kuipers E, Garety P, Fowler D et al, The London–East Anglia randomised controlled trial of cognitive-behavioural therapy for psychosis. I. Effects of the treatment phase. *Br J Psychiatry* 1997; **171**:319–327.

10. Wahlbeck K, Cheine M, Essali MA, Clozapine versus typical neuroleptic medication for schizophrenia. *Cochrane Database Syst Rev* 2000; **2**:CD000059.
11. Garety P, Kuipers E, Fowler D, Freeman D, Bebbington P, A cognitive model of the positive symptoms of psychosis. *Psychol Med* 2001; **31**:189–195.
12. Hemsley DR, A simple (or simplistic?) cognitive model for schizophrenia. *Behav Res Ther* 1993; **31**:633–645.
13. Frith CD, *The Cognitive Neuropsychology of Schizophrenia*. LEA Press: Hove, UK, 1992.
14. Kemp R, Kirov G, Everitt B, Hayward P, David A, Randomised controlled trial of compliance therapy: 18-month follow-up. *Br J Psychiatry* 1998; **172**:413–419.
15. Drury V, Birchwood M, Cochrane R, Macmillan F, Cognitive therapy and recovery from acute psychosis: a controlled trial. I. Impact on psychotic symptoms. *Br J Psychiatry* 1996; **169**:593–601.
16. Lewis S, Tarrier N, Haddock G et al, Randomised controlled trial of cognitive-behavioural therapy in early schizophrenia: acute-phase outcomes. *Br J Psychiatry* 2002; **181(Suppl 43)**:91–97.
17. Gumley A, O'Grady M, McNay L et al, Early intervention for relapse in schizophrenia: results of a randomised, controlled trial of cognitive behaviour therapy. *Psychol Med* 2003; **33**:419–431.
18. Yung A, Phillips LJ, McGorry PD et al, A step towards indicated prevention of schizophrenia. *Br J Psychiatry* 1998; **172(Suppl 33)**:14–20.
19. McGorry PD, Yung AR, Phillips LJ et al, Randomised controlled trial of interventions designed to reduce the risk of progression to first-episode psychosis in a clinical sample with subthreshold symptoms. *Arch Gen Psychiatry* 2002; **59**:921–928.
20. Morrison AP, Bentall RP, French P, Kilcommons A, Walford L, Lewis SW, A randomised controlled trial of early detection and cognitive therapy for preventing transition to psychosis in high risk individuals: study design and interim analysis of transition rate and psychological risk factors. *Br J Psychiatry* 2002; **181(Suppl 43)**:78–84.
21. Kay S, Fiszbein A, Opler LA, The positive and negative syndrome scale (PANSS) for schizophrenia. *Schizophr Bull* 1987; **13**:261–276.

chapter 19

Cognitive remediation is better than cognitive behaviour therapy

Til Wykes

The aim of this book is to try to challenge some of the assumptions held in psychiatry that may interfere with seeing the bigger picture. One belief currently held not only by the mental health community, but also now embodied in official guidance, is that only one individual psychological therapy, cognitive behaviour therapy (CBT), is the key to successful outcome and as such should be considered as part of the therapies offered to all patients. This information is now incorporated in both the UK National Institute for Clinical Excellence (NICE) schizophrenia guidelines and is being considered for the PORT guidelines in the USA. But is this really true? What about other sorts of therapy, particularly one new and innovative therapy for people with schizophrenia, cognitive remediation therapy (CRT)? This chapter will consider what we might expect from the two therapies and argues that even though cognitive remediation is in its infancy it is still likely to offer more advantages than CBT.

How do we measure outcome from psychological therapy for schizophrenia?

There are clearly two types of target. The primary one is the proximal target that the therapy is designed to affect; the secondary targets are usually theoretically linked to the primary targets but do not necessarily have a direct link to the therapy itself.

Both CBT and CRT, as their names suggest, are aimed at changing thinking, but they differ in their primary targets. The primary target for CBT is the symptom, so the main outcome is measured as a reduction in total symptoms, or perhaps as minor changes in the level of conviction of delusions. In contrast, the primary targets for CRT are the basic thinking skills themselves. They are thinking skills that are measured usually by formal neuropsychological tasks and are not related to emotionally meaningful material. My thesis is that these basic thinking skills are more important to the recovery of people with schizophrenia.

Cognition and schizophrenia

What all health professionals learn about schizophrenia is that cognition is important. Both Kraepelin and Bleuler included cognition as an important characteristic in their definitions of the disorder, even though they disagreed about the course of cognitive impairments. Not only is cognition important at the onset of the disorder, but cognitive disturbances are also clear in individuals who are vulnerable to the disorder prior to its onset.[1,2] We know that cognitive difficulties are present during episodes of the disorder and for some people they are also present between episodes of acute symptoms. The sorts of problems patients report are memory and attention problems (e.g. McGhie and Chapman[3]), mild reasoning biases (e.g. Garety[4]) and abnormal perceptions that are attributed as hallucinations and delusions (Maher and Spitzer[5]). These thinking skills problems are well known and documented in academic clinical research and are recognized by people with diagnoses of schizophrenia. There is therefore ample evidence that cognition is important in the disorder, but both types of therapy try to use cognition in different ways in order to aid recovery.

What is recovery?

The best people to ask what elements constitute recovery are the people who have the disorder. They say:

- I want to have a job;
- I want to have friends;
- I want to cook and eat when I want to; and
- I want to live in my own home and not in a hostel.

Clinical academics call these things vocational functioning, social functioning, life skills and dependence on psychiatric services. These recovery outcomes can be affected by rehabilitation and so each will be subject to a brief review about what the relation is between cognitive difficulties, symptoms and treatment in order to identify if symptoms or cognitive difficulties affect the outcome of treatment.

Vocational functioning

What is of interest in vocational functioning is evidence of the effects of symptoms and cognitive difficulties on treatment outcome. It is therefore important to investigate vocational rehabilitation services that have good outcomes to provide a stringent test of any putative predictor variables. One good example is the programme at the Veterans' Administration Hospital in West Haven, USA. This programme aims to allow people the choice of different types of job and provides 'on-the-job support' as well as group and individual activities to improve work skills. Bell and colleagues[6] investigated the effects of cognition on outcome and found that the majority of variance in outcome (e.g. work quality, work habits, etc.) was accounted for by cognition and that symptoms were not significant predictors. In addition Bryson and Bell reported that 29% of the variance in the improvement of work skills in the same programme was accounted for by cognition.[7] Again, symptoms were not a significant predictor. Cognition in both studies was measured with memory, attention and concentration tests.

Social functioning

For social functioning, Smith and colleagues[8] reported an interesting study of the recovery of patients following an acute admission. They measured social functioning improvements at intervals for 12 months and found that those with a good working memory improved their social functioning over the 12 months by about 20% on an observer-rated scale. However, those with poor working memory did not improve on the same scale. Positive symptoms at the time of admission did not account for this difference in social functioning recovery. The assumption is that following an acute admission patients will be provided with multiple treatments to improve recovery, so again cognition seems to be an impediment to change following treatment. This is a further replication of studies, e.g. Mueser et al,[9] which show that verbal memory difficulties impede learning from social skills training programmes.

Life skills

The ability to care for oneself, or life skills, was investigated in a study by Velligan and colleagues.[10] They showed that a composite measure of cognition accounted for 42% of the variances in life skills outcome after 18 months, and that symptoms could be dropped from the path model without losing explanatory power.

Dependence on psychiatric care

The last category of recovery is dependence on psychiatric care, which was investigated in a series of studies by myself and colleagues before and after the closure of a large psychiatric hospital, Netherne, in the UK. This hospital had a good reputation for psychiatric rehabilitation and its closure meant that even further efforts were made to place people in the least dependent psychiatric care. The series of studies investigated the effects of thinking flexibility, symptoms and social functioning as possible predictors of outcome over a 6-year period. In every analysis cognitive skill was an important predictor and at 6 years the variables that predicted 60% of the variances were cognition and previous skills. Again, symptoms did not contribute to the prediction model.

These studies are examples from the increasing corpus of data showing the importance of thinking skills in the process of recovery (e.g. Green et al[11]). This relation also has implications for the cost of psychiatric care for those with cognitive difficulties. Wykes et al have shown that the costs of care for people with a moderate-to-severe cognitive impairment and schizophrenia are far higher than the costs for the whole population of patients with the same diagnosis from the same area.[12] These costs are not spread across categories of care but are mostly accounted for by the increased costs of residential and inpatient care. Given the data alluded to above even the best current rehabilitation programmes, which do improve overall outcome, will be hampered by problems with cognitive difficulties and therefore would be unlikely to reduce this cost burden significantly.

One option would be to provide specific therapy to improve cognition that would then remove the major impediment. Do we have a therapy that will help? One possibility would be CRT. The development of CRT is very different to that of most therapies. It emerged at a time when the scientific community thought, erroneously, that if there were no changes over time in a variable, i.e. cognition, then this variable was incapable of changing. The literature on the negative findings of CRT proliferated as editors were willing to publish data that fitted the current zeitgeist of extreme pessimism.

Can we change in cognition?

There was some scepticism about improving cognition. In 1992 the *Schizophrenia Bulletin* produced a section of commentaries in a special issue. These are two of the titles:

'Cognitive rehabilitation for schizophrenia: Is it possible? Is it necessary?'

(Bellack)[13]

'Cognitive remediation in schizophrenia: Proceed . . . with caution!'

(Hogarty and Flesher)[14]

The authors of both papers have overcome their scepticism and now have programmes of research on cognitive remediation. But doubt about its possible efficacy still exists and was recently fuelled by a strange meta-analysis[15] that informed the UK NICE guidelines. The authors suggested that 'the present results certainly do not justify the incorporation of cognitive remediation into clinical practice'. This conclusion was based on only five studies that differed considerably in the type of therapy, the time for therapy (1 day to 3 months) and the measurement of their outcome.

But is cognitive remediation therapy effective?

All the accumulated evidence, including the negative findings, has been very instructive as it has shown all the blind alleys that have been entered before more positive findings were found. We now know that there are a variety of methods that will help clinicians to improve people's thinking skills and their cognitive style. Table 19.1 shows the effects of some of the techniques

Table 19.1 Techniques for cognitive remediation therapy (CRT)[a]

Thinking skill	CRT type	Positive outcome
Attention	Endless Practice	No
	Individual CRT	Yes
	Group CRT	No
Memory	Endless computer practice	No
	Individual CRT	Yes
	Group CRT	Maybe
Flexibility	Computer practice	No
	Individual CRT	Yes
	Group CRT	Maybe
Problem solving	Computerized CRT	Yes

[a] Data from: Medalia et al;[16–18] Wykes et al;[12,19] Spaulding et al;[20,21] Bellack et al;[22] Bell et al;[6] Kurtz et al.[23]

that have been tested on specific targets. Endless practice does not seem to work for any cognitive target. Group CRT does not enjoy as much support as individual CRT. But in a recent meta-analysis of 12 trials Krabbendam and Aleman showed that the effect size of CRT on cognition was 0.45, and that those studies which used a particular technique of teaching strategies rather than using practice had a significant effect.[24]

Which is best the 'R' or the 'B'?

CRT does improve its primary target – cognition. Despite scepticism shown in other chapters in this book, CBT improves symptoms, its primary target. In a meta-analysis carried out by Wykes et al, the mean effect size from 18 trials was about 0.37 and all but one of the trials shows a positive effect.[25] So where primary targets are concerned we are neck and neck.

But CRT also improves symptoms. In a recent randomized controlled trial where symptoms were rated blind to group allocation it was shown that, when cognition improves, ratings of auditory hallucinations also improve (Figure 19.1).[12] Brain activation also changes. In a recent study of the effects of CRT using functional magnetic resonance imaging, activation of frontal regions increased in the CRT group during a working memory task.[26]

What are symptoms, the primary target of CBT, associated with? They are clearly correlated with admission to hospital and distress, so we need to know if CBT affects either of these. In terms of the number of admissions to

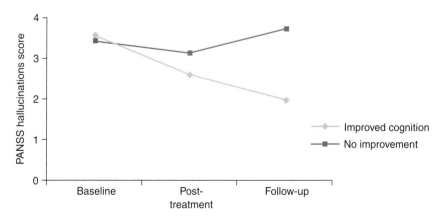

Figure 19.1 *The effect of cognitive improvements on auditory hallucinations. (From Wykes T et al.* Schizophr Res *2003;* **61:***163–174.[12])*

hospital, for CBT there is very little evidence that there is any effect on admission or on social functioning or on distress.

Do cognitive improvements get to the parts that cognitive behaviour therapy doesn't reach?

There are studies showing improvements in symptoms following CRT (e.g. Medalia et al[14]) as well as social functioning.[17] There is also some evidence that people who use CRT might go on to using more day care.[12] However, this may be considered as positive because, as the data show, it is not that more people were referred to day care, but that the people who were referred had a higher attendance rate. Individuals may then have the opportunity to benefit from the opportunities that these programmes offered.

One example of the way in which CRT does affect an individual comes from the therapy offered by our team. One older woman offered therapy had to have it provided in her own home as she never left the house (and rarely got out of bed). After 2 weeks she was able to attend a community health team to receive therapy accompanied by a carer. Within 6 weeks she began to attend on her own arriving earlier than the appointment time. Her close relatives reported that she now got out of bed not only on therapy days but on other days too and there was a marked improvement in her behaviour towards them.

These behaviour changes during therapy mirror the changes in self-esteem found during therapy but lost later.[12,19] Engagement with therapy has been reported by several authors as good with few dropouts during therapy.

The data currently available for CRT are sparse, whereas there are more large scale trials available for CBT. But the evidence for CRT is good, the latest trials clearly showing effects with clear messages for the type of therapy likely to provide these improvements. Both the primary targets of CBT and CRT are useful to change. However, in terms of likely secondary effects that service users give prominence to, and both the theoretical and empirical relations of cognition to these secondary targets, it appears that it is CRT that can change the patient's life and aid recovery. This does not mean that CBT should not be provided but that the two therapies should perhaps be seen as synergistic in a comprehensive psychological treatment programme.

References

1. David AS, Malmberg A, Brandt L, Allebeck P, Lewis G, IQ and risk for schizophrenia: a population-based cohort study. *Psychol Med* 1997; **27**:1311–1323.
2. Cannon M, Caspi A, Moffitt T et al, Evidence for early-childhood, pan-developmental impairment specific to schizophreniform disorder: results from a longitudinal birth cohort. *Arch Gen Psychiatry* 2002; **59**:449–456.
3. McGhie A, Chapman J, Disorders of attention and perception in early schizophrenia. *Br J Med Psychol* 1961; **34**:103–117.
4. Garety P, Reasoning and delusions. *Br J Psychiatry* 1991; **159 (Suppl 14)**:14–18.
5. Maher B, Spitzer M, Delusions. In: Costello CG (ed), *Symptoms of Schizophrenia.* pp. 92–120, Wiley: Chichester, 1993.
6. Bell M, Bryson G, Greig T, Corcoran C, Wexler B, Neurocognitive enhancement therapy with work therapy: effects on neurocognitive test performance. *Arch Gen Psychiatry* 2001; **58**:763–768.
7. Bryson G, Bell M, Initial and final work performance in schizophrenia: cognitive and symptom predictors. *Journal of Nervous & Mental Disease* 2003; **191**:87–92.
8. Smith TE, Hull J, Huppert J, Silverstein SM, Recovery from psychosis in schizophrenia and schizoaffective disorder: symptoms and neurocognitive rate-limiters for the development of social behavior skills. *Schizophr Res* 2002; **55**:229–237.
9. Mueser KT, Bellack AS, Douglas MS, Wade JH, Prediction of social skill acquisition in schizophrenic and major affective disorder patients from memory and symptomatology. *Psychiatry Res* 1991; **37**:281–296.
10. Velligan D, Mahurin R, Diamond P, Hazleton B, Eckert S, Miller A, The functional significance of symptomatology and cognitive function in schizophrenia. *Schizophr Res* 1997; **25**:21–31.
11. Green MF, Kern R, Braff D, Mintz J, Neurocognitive deficits and functional outcome in schizophrenia: are we measuring the 'right stuff'? *Schizophr Bull* 2000; **26**:119–136.
12. Wykes T, Reeder C, Williams C, Corner J, Rice C, Everitt B, Are the effects of cognitive remediation therapy (CRT) durable? Results from an exploratory trial. *Schizophr Res* 2003; **61**:163–174.
13. Bellack A, Cognitive rehabilitation for schizophrenia: Is it possible? Is it necessary? *Schizophr Bull* 1992; **18**:43–50.
14. Hogarty GE, Flesher S, Cognitive remediation in schizophrenia: proceed . . . with caution! *Schizophr Bull* 1992; **18**:51–57.
15. Pilling S, Bebbington P, Kuipers E et al, Psychological treatments in schizophrenia: II. Meta-analyses of randomized controlled trials of social skills training and cognitive remediation. *Psychol Med* 2002; **32**:783–791.
16. Medalia A, Aluma M, Tryon W, Merriam A, Effectiveness of attention training in schizophrenia. *Schizophr Bull* 1998; **24**:147–152.
17. Medalia A, Revheim N, Casey M, Remediation of memory disorders in schizophrenia. *Psychol Med* 2001; **30**:1451–1459.
18. Medalia A, Revheim N, Casey M, The remediation of problem-solving skills in schizophrenia. *Schizophr Bull* 2001; **27**:259–267.
19. Wykes T, Reeder C, Corner J, Williams C, Everitt B, The effects of neurocognitive remediation on executive processing in patients with schizophrenia. *Schizophr Bull* 1999; **25**:291–307.
20. Spaulding W, Reed D, Storzbach D, Sullivan M, Weiler M, Richardson C, The effects of a remediational approach to cognitive therapy for schizophrenia. In: Wykes T, Tarrier N, Lewis S (eds), *Outcome and Innovation in Psychological Treatment of Schizophrenia.* pp. 145–160, Wiley: Chichester, 1998.

21. Spaulding W, Fleming Shelley K, Reed D, Sullivan M, Storzbach D, Lam M, Cognitive functioning in schizophrenia: implications for psychiatric rehabilitation. *Schizophr Bull* 1999; **25**:275–289.
22. Bellack A, Weinhardt L, Gold J, Gearon J, Generalization of training effects in schizophrenia. *Schizophr Res* 2001; **48**:255–262.
23. Kurtz MM, Moberg PJ, Gur RC, Gur RE, Approaches to cognitive remediation of neuropsychological deficits in schizophrenia: a review and meta-analysis. *Neuropsychol Rev* 2001; **11**:197–210.
24. Krabbendam L, Aleman A, Cognitive rehabilitation in schizophrenia: a quantitative analysis of controlled studies. *Psychopharmacology* 2003; (in press).
25. Wykes T, Tarrier N, Everitt B, Cognitive behaviour therapy (CBT) for schizophrenia: effect sizes, clinical models and methodological rigour. 2003; (in preparation)
26. Wykes T, Brammer M, Mellers J et al, Effects on the brain of a psychological treatment: cognitive remediation therapy (CRT): functional magnetic resonance imaging in schizophrenia. *Br J Psychiatry* 2002; **181**:144–152.

chapter 20

The shared genetic architecture which underlies schizophrenia and bipolar disorder

Elvira Bramon and Pak Sham

Competing models for psychosis

The orthodox view that psychotic disorders can be divided into schizophrenia and bipolar disease stems from extensive clinical observations by Emil Kraepelin in the early years of the twentieth century.[1] Current psychiatric nosology, whether American or European, classifies schizophrenia and bipolar disorder as two distinct diagnostic categories, with presumed independent aetiologies, and any clinical overlap at the patient or family levels tends to be attributed to diagnostic misclassification.

An alternative view, which mirrors the pre-Kraepelinean position of unitary psychosis, is that different forms of psychosis represent a continuum of disorders, with schizophrenia at the most severe end of the spectrum.[2] This dimensional approach could easily account for the striking clinical, neurobiological and epidemiological similarities between schizophrenia and bipolar disorder.

More recently, the orthodox and continuum views of psychosis have been challenged by a model based on aetiological overlap. If schizophrenia and bipolar disorder are multifactorial diseases, with common risk factors, some degree of aetiological overlap should not be surprising. Under a liability-threshold formulation of this model, one would expect the liability for the two disorders to be correlated rather than independent. Thus, as shown in Figure 20.1, a plot of liabilities for the two disorders would give an elliptical

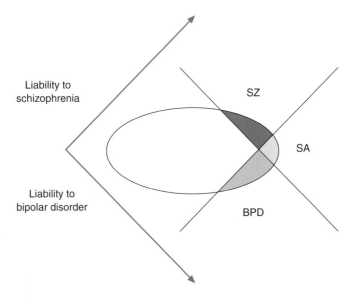

Figure 20.1 *Dimensions of liability to schizophrenia (SZ), bipolar disorder (BPD) and schizo-affective (SA) disorder.*

shape. Individuals exceeding liability thresholds in either axis would develop schizophrenia or bipolar disorder respectively and those who exceeded liability thresholds for both disorders would emerge with a schizo-affective diagnosis. But what is the evidence for there being a shared genetic liability or at least a partial sharing?

Evidence from epidemiological, family and twin studies

Overlap of risk factors

Schizophrenia and bipolar disorder display considerable overlap not only in phenomenology and epidemiology but also in risk factors. Van Os and colleagues argued for a dimensional view by pointing out that there is little evidence of any risk factor being specific to any diagnostic category within the functional psychoses.[3] Obstetric complications, consistently reported as a risk factor for schizophrenia, are also more prevalent among patients with affective disorders than controls. The same can be said of minor physical anomalies and dermatoglyphic abnormalities. Childhood adjustment deficits have been reported in patients with depression and bipolar disorder. The season-of-birth effect for schizophrenia and the role of prenatal infections have also been reported in bipolar disorder, especially for those cases with mania. Finally, cerebral ventricle enlargements, although less marked than in schizophrenia, are also present in affective psychosis.[4]

Is there familial co-aggregation between psychotic and affective disorders?

Family studies have consistently shown that the first-degree relatives of probands with schizophrenia are at increased risk for schizophrenia, schizo-affective disorder and schizotypal personality disorder. Similarly, family studies have also revealed that first-degree relatives of bipolar probands have an increased risk to develop bipolar disorder, schizo-affective disorder and unipolar depression.[5] However, whether there is increased cross-disorder familial risk for bipolar disorder or schizophrenia has been controversial.

Inadequate sample size and statistical power may have contributed to this confusion. The familial aggregation of schizophrenia with itself is expected to be greater than its co-aggregation with bipolar disorder, and most studies were powered to detect familial aggregation of schizophrenia with itself or bipolar disorder with itself but not their co-aggregation.

The largest family study to date used the Swedish inpatient register and pooled over 13 000 and 5 000 cases with schizophrenia and bipolar disorder, respectively (Table 20.1). Cross-disorder incidence ratios were clearly increased for both full and half siblings, providing unequivocal evidence for familial co-aggregation between schizophrenia and bipolar disorder.[6] Sceptics will however argue that this finding may be due to diagnostic misclassification.

Table 20.1 The Swedish inpatient register study. Strong evidence for familial co-aggregation[6]

Probands	Standardized incidence ratios			
	Full Sibs		Half Sibs	
	SZ	BPD	SZ	BPD
SZ (13 870)	7.4	3.6	4.4	2.8
BPD (5400)	4.4	12.8	2.2	8.1

SZ, schizophrenia; BPD, bipolar disorder.

Evidence from twin research and model fitting

In the classical study by Slater and Shields[7] the siblings of index twins with schizophrenia showed a similar prevalence of affective disorder and schizophrenia, while their parents were more likely to suffer affective disorder than schizophrenia. A curious case of identical triplets, two diagnosed with schizophrenia and the third with bipolar disorder, highlighted how the same genetic makeup could result in diverse forms of psychosis.[8] More recently, data from the Maudsley twin series (Figure 20.2) showed that cross-diagnostic concordance rates were greatly increased for monozygotic twins and modest for dizygotics. In addition, using model fitting techniques, common as well as diagnosis-specific genetic contributions to the variance in liability to schizophrenia and mania were found. However, diagnosis-specific genetic effects for schizo-affective disorder were negligible. The above twin analyses are in favour of a significant overlap in the genes contributing to schizo-

Proband	77 MZ Co-twins			89 DZ Co-twins		
	SZ	SA	Mania	SZ	SA	Mania
SZ	**40.8**	8.2	8.2	**5.3**	5.3	0
SA	26.1	**39.1**	26.1	4.5	**4.5**	0
Mania	13.6	31.8	**36.4**	3.7	3.7	**7.4**

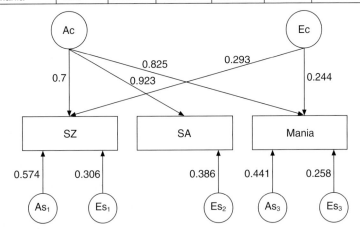

Figure 20.2 *The Maudsley twin series. The table shows cross-diagnostic probandwise concordance rates. The path diagram models the genetic and environmental influences to psychotic disorders. Ac/Ec, genetic/environmental influences common to the three diagnoses; As/Es, genetic/environmental effects specific to each diagnosis; MZ, monozygotic; DZ, dizygotic; SZ, schizophrenia; SA, Schizo-affective disorder.*

phrenia, schizo-affective disorder and mania.[9] However, in an alternative interpretation by Kendler,[10] genetic factors influencing risk for mania may not necessarily be the same in people with or without a comorbid diagnosis of schizophrenia. While modelling of phenotypic measures reaches increasing complexity, definitive answers will ultimately require evidence from molecular genetics.

Evidence from molecular research

Both schizophrenia and bipolar disorder have high heritability with estimates around 80%.[9,11] Given the evidence for overlap in familial susceptibility for bipolar and schizophrenic disorders, could this overlap be of genetic origin? If so, molecular genetic studies should report loci in common.

Genome-wide scans: can meta-analyses clarify the confusion?

Over the past 20 years numerous genome scans have been undertaken searching for susceptibility genes for both schizophrenia and bipolar disorder and their inconsistent findings have generated some confusion. Again as a result of power limitations, few studies exceed genome-wide significance levels and attempts to replicate a specific finding require even larger samples. Faced with these problems, Badner and Gershon conducted a meta-analysis of all published genome-wide scans and identified the most significant linkages for schizophrenia and bipolar disorder.[12] The remarkable result was that two zones (13q and 22q) showed strong evidence of linkage for both disorders. The authors concluded that these two regions were likely to harbour susceptibility loci common to bipolar disorder as well as schizophrenia. A subsequent collaborative meta-analysis of genome scans also identified a number of candidate regions for either schizophrenia[13] or bipolar disorder[14] but found no overlap of susceptibility regions between the two disorders (Table 20.2).

The conflicting results between two meta-analyses published only a year apart may be due to differences in statistical methodology and in the selection of datasets. Badner and Gershon included all published studies until mid-2002, regardless of their size. Instead, the collaborative meta-analyses pooled published data as well as conference presentations and personal communications, but excluded small studies.[12–14]

In addition to the above controversies, there is a further challenge in that genomic regions covered by linkage techniques are large and therefore some

Table 20.2 Meta-analyses of genome-wide scans

Meta-analysis	Schizophrenia	Bipolar disorder	Main conclusions
Badner and Gershon (2002)[12a]	8p (MM 50) 13q (MM 85) 22q (MM 32)	13q (MM 79) 22q (MM 36)	13q (MM 85) and 22q (MM 36) were highly significant and common to bipolar disorder and schizophrenia.
Collaborative meta-analyses			
Lewis et al (2003)[13] for the studies on schizophrenia	2p12-q22.1	9p22.3-21.1 10q11.21-22.1 14q24.1-32.12	No regions with significant linkage were found to be common to both disorders. Of note, 8p showed significant linkage with schizophrenia in both meta-analyses.
Segurado et al (2003)[14] for the studies on bipolar disorder	5q, 3p, 11q, 6p, 1q, 22q, 8p, 20q, 14p, 16q, 18q, 10p, 15q, 6q, 17q	9p, 18p-q, 14q, 8q	

[a](MM) indicate the location according to the Marshfield map.
Regions with highly significant linkage ($P < 0.01$) are in bold. All other regions reported were
significant at the 5% level.

overlap in the linkage zone does not necessarily imply that the same genes are involved in both disorders. The unequivocal confirmation of genetic overlap would require evidence of association between a specific marker and both schizophrenia and bipolar disorder.

Are there any common loci for psychotic and mood disorders? – Association studies

As reviewed by Harrison and Owen, studies of candidate genes such as catechol-*O*-methyltransferase (*COMT*), proline dehydrogenase (*PRODH*), G-protein signalling 4 (*RGS4*) and the α-7 nicotinic acetylcholine receptor gene (*CHRNA7*) have yielded interesting but inconclusive evidence for association with schizophrenia.[15] Many of these candidate genes have yet to be examined in bipolar disorder.

As for the association between *COMT* and bipolar disorder, after a few studies providing both positive and negative findings,[16] interest seemed to fade. An association between *COMT* and schizophrenia has been reported,[17] and although this has not been replicated, a recent study has found an interesting effect of *COMT* on frontal lobe function.[18]

Brain derived neurotrophic factor (BDNF) is thought to be involved in synaptic development, particularly in dopaminergic and serotonergic pathways, and its expression can be influenced by antidepressant medication. Except for Muglia and colleagues,[19] who advocated *BDNF* to be a gene predisposing to schizophrenia, five previous association studies were negative. Instead, they are beginning to show that the *BDNF* gene may play a role in the pathogenesis of bipolar and schizoaffective disorders, and even possibly depression; although this requires further replication.[20] *BDNF* is therefore a promising, yet still controversial, candidate gene to be shared by psychotic and mood disorders.

Systematic association screening of positive linkage regions has recently identified susceptibility genes for schizophrenia. Of these, *neuregulin* (*NRG1*) and *dysbindin* are the most strongly supported loci.[15,21,22] It is now of great interest to investigate whether these two schizophrenia loci might also be involved in bipolar disorder and findings can be expected imminently. Similarly, by following up the chromosomal 13 linkage region, Chumakov and colleagues reported a significant association between the *G72* and *G30* genes with schizophrenia, and a possible interaction with the D-amino acid oxidase (*DAAO*) gene on chromosome 12.[23] The authors highlighted the

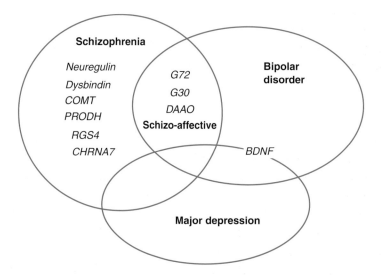

Figure 20.3 *Proposed susceptibility genes for psychotic and mood disorders. COMT, catechol-O-Methyltransferase; PRODH, proline dehydrogenase; RGS4, G-protein signalling 4; CHRNA7, α-7 nicotinic acetylcholine receptor. (Modified from Kennedy J. In:* Bipolar Disorder: The Upswing in Research and Treatment, *2003.[25])*

involvement of *N*-methyl-D-aspartate receptor regulation pathways in schizophrenia. Interestingly, Hattori and colleagues recently replicated the association of the same *G72/G30* genes to bipolar disorder in two independent pedigree series.[24] Thus, in agreement with the linkage evidence for the 13q region, these association analyses suggest that susceptibility loci exist in the vicinity of the *G72/G30* genes for both schizophrenia and bipolar disorder. This constitutes the first direct demonstration of shared gene(s) conveying risk for both disorders. Figure 20.3 is a speculative diagram of the roles of various genes currently thought to be involved in the psychoses.

Conclusion

After nearly a hundred years the Kraepelinian dichotomy is being increasingly challenged. Susceptibility genes have been identified and replicated for schizophrenia and similar progress can be expected in bipolar disorder. The elucidation of susceptibility genes, whether specific or shared across diagnoses, will finally resolve the controversies over the nosology of psychoses.

References

1. Kraepelin E, *Dementia Praecox, Paraphrenia*. Livingstone: Edinburgh, 1919.
2. Crow TJ, The continuum of psychosis and its implication for the structure of the gene. *Br J Psychiatry* 1986; **149**:419–429.
3. Van Os J, Gilvarry C, Bale R et al, A comparison of the utility of dimensional and categorical representations of psychosis. *Psychol Med* 1999; **29**:595–606.
4. McDonald C, Bullmore E, Sham P et al, Genetic risks for schizophrenia and bipolar disorder are associated with specific (grey) and generic (white) brain structural phenotypes (Submitted for publication).
5. Taylor M, Are schizophrenia and affective disorder related? A selective literature review. *Am J Psychiatry* 1992; **149**:22–32.
6. Osby U, Brandt L, Terenius L, The risk for schizophrenia and bipolar disorder in siblings to probands with schizophrenia and bipolar disorder. *Am J Medical Genet* 2001; **105**:O56.
7. Slater E, Shields J, *Psychotic and Neurotic Illneses in Twins*. Medical Research Council Special Report 278. Her Majesty's Stationery Office: London, 1953.
8. McGuffin P, Reveley A, Holland A, Identical triplets – non-identical psychosis. *Br J Psychiatry* 1982; **140**:1–6.
9. Cardno AG, Rijsdijk FV, Sham PC, Murray RM, McGuffin P, A twin study of genetic relationships between psychotic symptoms. *Am J Psychiatry* 2002; **159**:539–545.
10. Kendler KS, Hierarchy and heritability: the role of diagnosis and modeling in psychiatric genetics. *Am J Psychiatry* 2002; **159**:515–518.
11. McGuffin P, Rijsdijk F, Andrew M, Sham P, Katz R, Cardno A, The heritability of

bipolar affective disorder and the genetic relationship to unipolar depression. *Arch Gen Psychiatry* 2003; **60**:497–502.

12. Badner JA, Gershon ES, Meta-analysis of whole-genome linkage scans of bipolar disorder and schizophrenia. *Mol Psychiatry* 2002; **7**:405–411.

13. Lewis CM, Levinson DF, Wise LH et al, Genome scan meta-analysis of schizophrenia and bipolar disorder, part II: Schizophrenia. *Am J Human Genet* 2003; **73**:34–48.

14. Segurado R, Detera-Wadleigh SD, Levinson DF et al, Genome scan meta-analysis of schizophrenia and bipolar disorder, Part III: bipolar disorder. *Am J Hum Genet* 2003; **73**:49–62.

15. Harrison PJ, Owen MJ, Genes for schizophrenia? Recent findings and their pathophysiological implications. *Lancet* 2003; **361**:417–419.

16. Gutierrez B, Bertranpetit J, Guillamat R et al, Association analysis of the catechol-*O*-methyltransferase gene and bipolar affective disorder. *Am J Psychiatry* 1997; **154**:113–115.

17. Li T, Ball D, Zhao J et al, Family-based linkage disequilibrium mapping using SNP marker haplotypes: application to a potential locus for schizophrenia at chromosome 22q11. *Mol Psychiatry* 2000; **5**:77–84.

18. Goldberg TE, Egan MF, Gscheidle T et al, Executive subprocesses in working memory – Relationship to catechol-*O*-methyltransferase Val158Met genotype and schizophrenia. *Arch Gen Psychiatry* 2003; **60**:889–896.

19. Muglia P, Vicente AM, Verga M, King N, Macciardi F, Kennedy JL, Association between the BDNF gene and schizophrenia. *Mol Psychiatry* 2003; **8**:146–147.

20. Neves-Pereira M, Mundo E, Muglia P, King N, Macciardi F, Kennedy JL, The brain-derived neurotrophic factor gene confers susceptibility to bipolar disorder: Evidence from a family-based association study. *Am J Hum Genet* 2002; **71**:651–655.

21. Stefansson H, Sarginson J, Kong A et al, Association of neuregulin 1 with schizophrenia confirmed in a Scottish population. *Am J Hum Genet* 2003; **72**:83–87.

22. Schwab SG, Knapp M, Mondabon S et al, Support for association of schizophrenia with genetic variation in the 6p22.3 gene, dysbindin, in sib-pair families with linkage and in an additional sample of triad families. *Am J Hum Genet* 2003; **72**:185–190.

23. Chumakov I, Blumenfeld M, Guerassimenko O et al, Genetic and physiological data implicating the new human gene G72 and the gene for D-amino acid oxidase in schizophrenia. *Proc Nat Acad Sci USA* 2002; **99**:13675–13680.

24. Hattori E, Liu CY, Badner JA et al, Polymorphisms at the *G72/G30* gene locus, on 13q33, are associated with bipolar disorder in two independent pedigree series. *Am J Hum Genet* 2003; **72**:1131–1140.

25. Kennedy JL, Now that we have some genes (in Toronto at least). In: *Bipolar Disorder: The Upswing in Research and Treatment*. Institute of Psychiatry, King's College: London, 2003.

chapter 21

Are there structural brain differences between schizophrenia and bipolar disorder?

Colm McDonald

For much of the century since Kraepelin divided psychotic illness into dementia praecox and manic depressive insanity (later to become known as schizophrenia and bipolar disorder), there has been controversy over whether these two disorders are really distinct from each other. Although the illnesses appear clinically distinguishable in their pure forms, there are no pathognomic symptoms on which clinicians can rely to differentiate them and discriminant function analysis of clinical data has failed to find a 'point of rarity' between the two disorders. Many patients with schizophrenia have symptoms of depression and mania; patients with bipolar disorder can have Schneiderian 'first rank' symptoms of schizophrenia during illness exacerbation; and the diagnosis of 'schizo-affective disorder' is necessary to categorize the significant fraction (around 8%) of psychotic patients who cannot be classified into either of the major psychotic branches.

Overlapping risk factors

Research in genetics has further blurred the line of demarcation between the illnesses. Family studies have consistently found higher rates of schizoaffective disorder, as well as unipolar depression, both in first-degree relatives of patients with schizophrenia and in first-degree relatives of patients with bipolar disorder. There is less evidence of direct coaggregation of schizophrenia and bipolar disorder in families, however, this may be due to lack of statistical power in some studies, as elaborated in Chapter 20. Furthermore the evidence for direct coaggregation becomes more substantial when data are confined to the more severe and psychotic forms of bipolar disorder rather than mild bipolar disorder.[1–3] Interestingly within bipolar disorder families, there is evidence for aggregation of psychotic symptoms,[4,5] also consistent with the hypothesis that a tendency to psychosis is genetically transmitted.

Several studies have also suggested overlapping epidemiological and neurobiological risk factors for the two illnesses. There is a well-replicated small excess of winter/spring births among those who go on to develop schizophrenia in adulthood and this excess has also been found for bipolar disorder.[6] Both disorders have an excess of onset in the summer months.[7] Cognitive, motor and social deficits have been identified by well-designed prospective trials in individuals who later go on to develop schizophrenia.[8] Although subjects who later develop bipolar disorder seem to have preservation of cognitive and motor skills, deficits in emotional and interpersonal skills are risk factors for both forms of psychosis.[9] Dermatoglyphic abnormalities are found in excess in schizophrenia and have also been reported in subjects with bipolar disorder.[10] Abnormalities of auditory-evoked potentials such as decreased amplitude and increased latency of the P300 wave are well known to be associated with schizophrenia, and bipolar disorder subjects are also reported to display increased P300 latency.[11] This chapter will consider whether the illnesses share brain structural deviations.

Structural magnetic resonance imaging studies

Despite heterogeneous patient samples and methodologies, neuroimaging studies consistently identify subtle volumetric deviations in a range of brain structures when schizophrenic patients are compared with controls. The nature of structural brain changes in bipolar disorder is far less certain. This is partially because there are over 250 neuroimaging studies published in schizophrenia but only about 40 in bipolar disorder. Furthermore, samples of individuals with bipolar disorder are often particularly heterogeneous, frequently encompassing global 'affective disorder' (which includes unipolar depressive illness) or 'affective psychosis' (including psychotic depression as well as bipolar affective disorder with psychotic features). There is evidence that the structural brain changes associated with unipolar depression differ from those associated with bipolar disorder, so collapsing these groups may not be valid. For example, there are reports of reduced volume of the hippocampus and basal ganglia in unipolar depression,[12,13] but the volumes of these structures appear to be preserved or enlarged when pure samples of bipolar disorder are examined.[14,15]

A summary of findings from volumetric magnetic resonance imaging (MRI) studies is provided in Table 21.1. Enlargement of the lateral and third ventricles is the most prominent finding in schizophrenia – a recent meta-analysis of 58 MRI studies reported a 26% enlargement of ventricular volume.[16] Although considerable evidence exists for ventricular enlargement in unipolar depression, especially among elderly individuals, reports are more variable for bipolar disorder.[17] Certainly any ventricular enlargement is less prominent than that found in schizophrenia and may be more apparent in those with more severe illness as indicated by the presence of psychotic symptoms, multiple episodes of illness or bipolar 1 compared with bipolar 2 disorder.[18–20] Third-ventricular enlargement is consistently reported in schizophrenia with most of the few studies which have examined this structure in bipolar disorder also reporting enlargement.

Schizophrenia is associated with a subtle reduction in global cerebral volume, of approximately 3% in magnitude, but cerebral volume tends to be preserved in bipolar disorder.[17] Over and above the global cerebral volume reduction in schizophrenia, there are further relative volume reductions in the frontal lobes, especially the dorsolateral prefrontal cortex. While most studies of unipolar depression report reduced frontal lobe volume, again the

Table 21.1 Volumetric changes in schizophrenia and bipolar disorder from magnetic resonance imaging studies

	Schizophrenia	Bipolar disorder
Cerebral volume	↓	↔
Lateral ventricles	↑	? ↑
Third ventricle	↑	? ↑
Prefrontal regions	↓	? ↓
Temporal lobe	↓	↔
Hippocampus	↓	↔
Amygdala	↓	↑
Thalamus	↓	? ↑
Basal ganglia	? ↑	↔
White matter hyperintensities	? ↑	↑

picture is less clear for pure bipolar disorder samples, with both positive and negative results reported. The prefrontal cortex consists of many functionally distinct regions and it may be that pathology is confined to certain subsections. Two of the three published studies which have examined the subgenual prefrontal cortex in bipolar disorder, a region known to have a role in regulating normal mood, have reported reductions in volume.[21,22]

Reduction in temporal lobe volume is well characterized in schizophrenia, especially of medial temporal lobe structures (including the hippocampus, amygdala and parahippocampal gyrus), and of the left superior temporal gyrus. The hippocampus forms a vital part of the memory system, which is impaired in schizophrenia, and some studies have correlated hippocampal volume reduction with memory impairment in schizophrenic subjects. There are several reports of hippocampal volume reduction in unipolar depression, which appears more prominent with repeated episodes of illness. The hippocampus is a major feedback site for glucocorticoids and it may be that hippocampal volume reduction is related to hypercortisolaemia, which also characterizes depression. However, there is little consistent evidence for volume reduction of temporal lobes or temporal subregions in bipolar disorder, including the hippocampus. Indeed there are now four published studies reporting enlarged volume of the amygdala in bipolar disorder.[23] This is in stark contrast to schizophrenia where this structure is reduced in volume. The amygdala (Figure 21.1) is closely connected to other limbic,

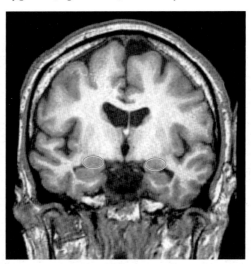

Figure 21.1 *Location of the amygdala in the medial temporal lobe on a T1-weighted coronal MRI scan.*

thalamic, basal ganglia and prefrontal regions which are involved in regulating mood and appears to have a role in organizing the autonomic and behavioural responses associated with emotion. It is unknown whether this enlargement of the amygdala is a trait feature that contributes to illness onset, or whether the amygdala undergoes hypertrophy with repeated manic episodes.

Relative thalamic volume reduction of around 4% over cerebral volume reduction is reported in schizophrenia,[16] with no evidence for thalamic reduction in bipolar disorder and two studies reporting increase in volume.[15] The basal ganglia are often slightly enlarged in schizophrenia. This structure is rich in dopaminergic input and the increased volume is usually attributed to the use of conventional antipsychotic medication, which potently blocks dopamine receptors, since it is not found in individuals who have had minimal antipsychotic treatment and the volume decreases on switching to an atypical antipsychotic.[24] Most studies in bipolar disorder have found no difference in the volume of basal ganglia structures compared with controls, with two studies reporting enlarged volume.[15]

One of the more consistent structural anomalies that is reported in bipolar disorder (in 80% of studies) is a qualitatively rated phenomenon: hyper-intensities within the periventricular and deep white matter which are observable on T2-weighted MRI images (Figure 21.2).[25] These lesions are also found in normal ageing, comorbid medical conditions (especially of vascular origin) and unipolar depression, but have been reported in excess even in

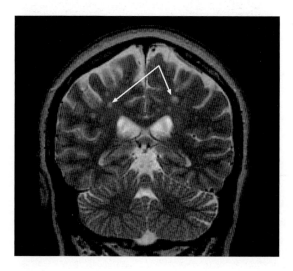

Figure 21.2 White matter hyperintensities (arrows) on a T2-weighted coronal MRI image.

young and first-onset bipolar subjects.[26,27] Their pathophysiology is unknown, although suggestions include infarction, atherosclerosis, arteriolar hyalinization, astrogliosis and demyelination. They have been investigated less extensively in schizophrenia, with some studies also finding high rates of such lesions, especially among elderly subjects with late onset of psychotic symptoms, although results have been mixed.[28]

Maudsley Family Study of Psychosis

Direct comparisons between schizophrenia and bipolar disorder or against the same control group are uncommon in the studies conducted to date. The Maudsley Family Study of Psychosis is a large study of neurobiological measures, including structural MRI analyses, of patients with schizophrenia and their unaffected relatives. More recently we have also collected a sample of bipolar subjects and their unaffected relatives from multiply-affected families. These subjects were selected to form a relatively homogeneous group, since all the bipolar patients had severe illness, fulfilling DSM-IV criteria for bipolar 1 disorder, and also had experienced psychotic symptoms at some stage of their illness. We hypothesized that such subjects would be most likely to share neurobiological abnormalities with schizophrenia. Volumetric MRI measurements of patients with schizophrenia (n = 41) or bipolar disorder (n = 37) were compared with normal subjects (n = 52). Whereas subjects with schizophrenia had significantly enlarged lateral ventricles ($P = 0.02$), third ventricle ($P = 0.01$) and cerebrospinal fluid spaces ($P = 0.03$), and reduced volume of the right hippocampus ($P = 0.03$), compared with controls, the bipolar patients did not significantly differ from the control group with regard to any of these measures. The results indicated that the most typical structural anomalies associated with schizophrenia are not found even in severe psychotic bipolar illness. These analyses were based on region of interest techniques where each structure of interest is painstakingly outlined and the analyses are confined to the relatively few structures chosen for measurement. Using computational morphometry, fully automated voxel-based techniques adapted from functional imaging, we also searched for volume deviation throughout the entire brain in an exploratory non-hypothesis-based analysis. When compared with controls, patients with schizophrenia had extensive regions of reduced grey matter volume involving the left dorsolateral prefrontal and orbitofrontal cortex, bilateral medial temporal lobes, bilateral insula, bilateral thalamus, right anterior superior and middle temporal gyri, cerebellar hemispheres and cerebellar vermis (P = 0.003); however, compared with controls, patients with bipolar disorder had no significant grey matter changes at all.[29] Patients with schizophrenia had extensive volume deficit involving white matter (P = 0.006) in the left frontal lobe, extending into the genu of the corpus callosum, and right temporoparietal region. Bipolar patients also had extensive volume reduction of white matter (P = 0.006) in the right frontal region, extending into the genu of the corpus callosum, and bilateral temporoparietal regions, extending into the splenium of the corpus callosum. This study indicates that the morphological characteristics of schizophrenia and psychotic bipolar disorder are distinct but overlapping. Schizophrenia is characterized by prominent deficits in volume of the subcortical and frontotemporal cortical grey matter, whereas grey matter volume is preserved in psychotic bipolar disorder. However, both disorders are characterized by volume deficits of white matter which overlap in temporoparietal regions. These findings are consistent with a hypothesis whereby the features more specific to schizophrenia – greater neurodevelopmental compromise, cognitive deficits and negative symptoms – have their roots in cortical/subcortical pathology, whereas psychosis in general is characterized by compromised anatomical connectivity.

Conclusion

In summary, Kraepelin's seminal dichotomy is partially supported by structural MRI studies, since many of the morphometric characteristics of schizophrenia and bipolar disorder are distinct. Bipolar disorder is relatively under-researched and it may not be valid for MRI studies to combine samples of patients with unipolar and bipolar illness. The evidence available to date suggests that, whereas schizophrenia is associated with volumetric reduction of frontotemporal, limbic and thalamic regions, bipolar disorder is characterized by preservation of temporal lobe structures and perhaps even enlargement of the amygdala. Potential overlap in structural deviations appears to be confined to ventricular enlargement, volumetric reduction of some prefrontal regions and white matter pathology. Structural white matter changes are largely under-researched in psychiatric disorders due to inadequate techniques for parcellation in comparison with neocortical and subcortical structures, but will be investigated more thoroughly in the future due to advances in computational morphometry and diffusion tensor imaging. Such studies will further elucidate whether structural anomalies common to the major psychoses reside in white matter deficit.

References

1. Kendler KS, McGuire M, Gruenberg AM, O'Hare A, Spellman M, Walsh D, The Roscommon Family Study. IV. Affective illness, anxiety disorders, and alcoholism in relatives. *Arch Gen Psychiatry* 1993; **50**:952–960.
2. Erlenmeyer-Kimling L, Adamo UH, Rock D et al, The New York High-Risk Project. Prevalence and comorbidity of axis I disorders in offspring of schizophrenic parents at 25-year follow-up. *Arch Gen Psychiatry* 1997; **54**:1096–1102.
3. Valles V, van Os J, Guillamat R et al, Increased morbid risk for schizophrenia in families of in-patients with bipolar illness. *Schizophr Res* 2000; **42**:83–90.
4. Potash JB, Willour VL, Chiu YF et al, The familial aggregation of psychotic symptoms in bipolar disorder pedigrees. *Am J Psychiatry* 2001; **158**:1258–1264.
5. Schurhoff F, Szoke A, Meary A et al, Familial aggregation of delusional proneness in schizophrenia and bipolar pedigrees. *Am J Psychiatry* 2003; **160**:1313–1319.
6. Torrey EF, Miller J, Rawlings R, Yolken RH, Seasonality of births in schizophrenia and bipolar disorder: a review of the literature. *Schizophr Res* 1997; **28**:1–38.
7. Takei N, O'Callaghan E, Sham P, Glover G, Tamura A, Murray R, Seasonality of admissions in the psychoses: effect of diagnosis, sex, and age at onset. *Br J Psychiatry* 1992; **161**:506–511.
8. Jones P, Rodgers B, Murray R, Marmot M, Child development risk factors for adult schizophrenia in the British 1946 birth cohort. *Lancet* 1994; **344**:1398–1402.
9. Cannon M, Caspi A, Moffitt TE et al, Evidence for early-childhood pan-developmental impairment specific to schizophreniform disorder: results from a longitudinal birth cohort. *Arch Gen Psychiatry* 2002; **59**:449–457.
10. Jelovac N, Milicic J, Milas M, Dodig G, Turek S, Ugrenovic Z, Dermatoglyphic analysis in bipolar affective disorder and schizophrenia – 'continuum of psychosis' hypothesis corroborated? *Coll Antropol* 1999; **23**:589–595.
11. Souza VB, Muir WJ, Walker MT et al, Auditory P300 event-related potentials and neuropsychological performance in schizophrenia and bipolar affective disorder. *Biol Psychiatry* 1995; **37**:300–310.
12. Sheline YI, Wang PW, Gado MH, Csernansky JG, Vannier MW, Hippocampal atrophy in recurrent major depression. *Proc Natl Acad Sci USA* 1996; **93**:3908–3913.
13. Parashos IA, Tupler LA, Blitchington T, Krishnan KR, Magnetic-resonance morphometry in patients with major depression. *Psychiatry Res* 1998; **84**:7–15.
14. Pearlson GD, Barta PE, Powers RE et al, Ziskind-Somerfeld Research Award 1996. Medial and superior temporal gyral volumes and cerebral asymmetry in schizophrenia versus bipolar disorder. *Biol Psychiatry* 1997; **41**:1–14.
15. Strakowski SM, Del Bello MP, Sax KW et al, Brain magnetic resonance imaging of structural abnormalities in bipolar disorder. *Arch Gen Psychiatry* 1999; **56**:254–260.
16. Wright IC, Rabe-Hesketh S, Woodruff PWR, David AS, Murray RM, Bullmore ET, Meta-analysis of regional brain volumes in schizophrenia. *Am J Psychiatry* 2000; **157**:16–25.
17. Beyer JL, Krishnan KR, Volumetric brain imaging findings in mood disorders. *Bipolar Disord* 2002; **4**:89–104.
18. Kato T, Shioiri T, Murashita J, Hamakawa H, Inubushi T, Takahashi S, Phosphorus-31 magnetic resonance spectroscopy and ventricular enlargement in bipolar disorder. *Psychiatry Res* 1994; **55**:41–50.
19. Hauser P, Matochik J, Altshuler LL et al, MRI-based measurements of temporal

lobe and ventricular structures in patients with bipolar I and bipolar II disorders. *J Affect Disord* 2000; **60**:25–32.

20. Strakowski SM, DelBello MP, Zimmerman ME et al, Ventricular and periventricular structural volumes in first- versus multiple-episode bipolar disorder. *Am J Psychiatry* 2002; **159**:1841–1847.

21. Drevets WC, Price JL, Simpson JR Jr et al, Subgenual prefrontal cortex abnormalities in mood disorders. *Nature* 1997; **386**:824–827.

22. Hirayasu Y, Shenton ME, Salisbury DF et al, Subgenual cingulate cortex volume in first-episode psychosis. *Am J Psychiatry* 1999; **156**:1091–1093.

23. Brambilla P, Harenski K, Nicoletti M et al, MRI investigation of temporal lobe structures in bipolar patients. *J Psychiatr Res* 2003; **37**:287–295.

24. Chakos MH, Lieberman JA, Alvir J, Bilder R, Ashtari M, Caudate nuclei volumes in schizophrenic patients treated with typical antipsychotics or clozapine. *Lancet* 1995; **345**:456–457.

25. Altshuler LL, Curran JG, Hauser P, Mintz J, Denicoff K, Post R, T2 hyperintensities in bipolar disorder: magnetic resonance imaging comparison and literature meta-analysis. *Am J Psychiatry* 1995; **152**:1139–1144.

26. Botteron KN, Vannier MW, Geller B, Todd RD, Lee BC, Preliminary study of magnetic resonance imaging characteristics in 8- to 16-year-olds with mania. *J Am Acad Child Adolesc Psychiatry* 1995; **34**:742–749.

27. Strakowski SM, Woods BT, Tohen M, Wilson DR, Douglass AW, Stoll AL, MRI subcortical signal hyperintensities in mania at first hospitalization. *Biol Psychiatry* 1993; **33**:204–206.

28. Davis KL, Stewart DG, Friedman JI et al, White matter changes in schizophrenia: evidence for myelin-related dysfunction. *Arch Gen Psychiatry* 2003; **60**:443–456.

29. McDonald C, Chitnis XA, Bullmore ET, Suckling J, Murray RM, Structural brain deviations associated with schizophrenia and psychotic bipolar disorder assessed using computational morphometry. *Schizophr Res* 2003; **60**:201–202.

chapter 22

Functional neural abnormalities in schizophrenia and bipolar disorder: are they similar or different?

Mary L Phillips

Intact perception and experience of emotion is vital for survival in the social environment. There has been increasing interest in the examination of the neurobiological basis of emotion perception in humans and non-human primates, and increasing evidence for abnormalities in emotion perception in patients with psychiatric disorders, including schizophrenia and bipolar disorder. This had led to the conceptualization of psychiatric disorders in terms of specific abnormalities of emotion perception. In this chapter, a brief outline will therefore be presented of findings from studies employing a variety of techniques which have helped to increase understanding of the nature of the neural systems underlying normal emotion perception. Findings from studies will then be described which have provided evidence for specific abnormalities in these neural systems, distinguishing patients with schizophrenia from those with bipolar disorder.

Neural systems underlying normal emotion perception

Emotion perception can be understood in terms of three related processes (Figure 22.1):[1]

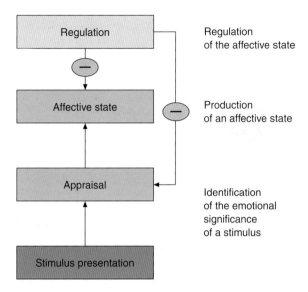

Figure 22.1 *The main processes important for emotion perception: (i) the identification of emotionally salient information; (ii) the generation of emotional experiences and behaviour in response to this information; and (iii) the regulation of these two processes so that the emotion is contextually appropriate.*

1. the identification and appraisal of emotionally salient information in the environment;
2. the generation of emotional experiences and behaviour in response to 1;
3. the regulation of emotional experiences and behaviour. This may involve an inhibition of processes 1 and 2 so that the affective state and behaviour generated in response to environmental stimuli are contextually appropriate.

Findings from studies which have increased understanding of the nature of the neural correlates of these processes, in particular processes 1 and 2, are outlined below.

Identification of emotionally salient information

A well-described 'limbic' circuit, including ventral regions of the anterior cingulate gyrus, ventromedial prefrontal cortex, ventral striatum and the dorsomedial nucleus of the thalamus, has been previously identified as potentially important for motivation and emotion processing (see Alexander et al[2]). Specific neural regions have also been highlighted as particularly important for the identification of emotional stimuli, however, and include the amygdala and anterior insula.[3]

The amygdala is a small, almond-shaped region within the anterior part of the temporal lobe. Several studies of non-human primates, of patients with amygdala lesions, and those employing functional neuroimaging techniques have demonstrated the importance of the amygdala in face and eye gaze identification,[4] the identification of emotional expressions displayed by others, in particular, threat-related emotions such as fear, but also sadness and happiness, and in the response to non-facial displays of emotion, including unpleasant auditory, olfactory and gustatory stimuli, and the memory for emotional information.[3] The insula is a part of the cerebral cortex at the base of the lateral fissure. Studies have demonstrated the role of the anterior (agranular) insula in particular in the autonomic response to aversive stimuli, fear reactivity and anticipatory anxiety, and in the identification of displays of disgust in others.[3]

Generation of emotional experiences and behaviours

Studies of non-human primates, patients with amygdala lesions and patients with temporal lobe epilepsy, in whom abnormal activation of the amygdala occurs, have indicated the role of the amygdala in the generation of appropriate emotional experiences and behaviours in response to emotionally salient, and, in particular, fearful stimuli.[3] Other studies using similar techniques have highlighted the role of the anterior insula in the generation of the response to aversive and disgust-provoking material. The anterior insula has been demonstrated to be important for conditioned taste aversion, unpleasant taste and pain perception, anxiety and nausea.[3]

Other regions involved in the response to emotionally salient material include the ventral region of the anterior cingulate gyrus and ventromedial and ventrolateral regions of the prefrontal cortex. The ventral anterior cingulate gyrus, including subgenual and pregenual or rostral regions, is important for autonomic function and emotional behaviour. Studies employing functional neuroimaging techniques in humans have demonstrated activity within this structure in mood induction and during anxiety associated with the anticipation of pain.[5] The ventromedial prefrontal cortex and the medial region of this structure, the orbitofrontal cortex, which has direct connections with the amygdala, appear to be particularly important in animals and humans for the perception of pleasant and unpleasant odours, flavours and tactile stimuli, the representation of the reward value of a stimulus and the way in which this representation then guides goal-directed and normal social behaviour.[6] The ventrolateral pre-frontal cortex lies lateral to the orbitofrontal cortex on the ventral surface of the frontal lobes. Human functional neuroimaging studies have demonstrated activity within this region during the response to emotional information, including the induction of sad mood and the recall of personal memories and emotional material (see Drevets[5]).

Regulation of emotional experiences and behaviour

To date, there is limited understanding of the neural basis of emotion regu-lation. There is, however, some indication, primarily from studies employing functional neuroimaging techniques in humans, for the role in this process of the hippocampus and a dorsal neural system, comprising dorsal regions of the anterior cingulate gyrus, dorsomedial and dorsolateral prefrontal cor-tices, structures important for selective attention, planning, motor responses to emotional stimuli, and the integration of these processes with emotional input (see Drevets[5] and Phillips et al[1]). Furthermore, recent evidence from neuroimaging studies has implicated the right superior/dorsomedial pre-frontal gyrus and the right dorsal anterior cingulate gyrus in the suppression of emotional states and arousal[7] (see Phillips et al[1]). Levesque et al have also reported orbitofrontal cortical activation during the voluntary suppression of emotional states and behaviour,[7] although this region has a predominant regulatory role in the mediation of autonomic states rather than voluntary inhibition of emotional behaviour per se.[1]

Summary

Overall, these findings indicate the involvement of a distributed ventral neural system, including the ventral striatum, specific thalamic nuclei, the amygdala and anterior insula, and ventromedial regions of the prefrontal cortex, in the perception of emotionally salient information. Whilst the ventral striatum, dorsomedial nucleus of the thalamus, amygdala and anterior insula appear to be important for the identification of emotionally salient stimuli, ventromedial and ventrolateral prefrontal cortical regions appear to be of particular importance for the generation of emotional experi-ences and behaviour in response to these stimuli. Dorsal prefrontal regions may have a particular role in the voluntary regulation of emotional behaviour (Figure 22.2).

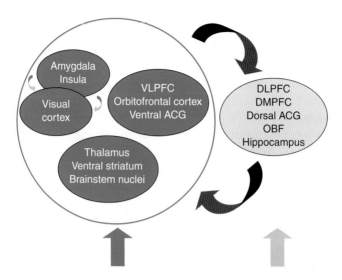

Figure 22.2 *Schematic diagram depicting neural structures important for the three processes related to emotion perception. Depicted in darker blue are the ventral striatum, dorsomedial nucleus of the thalamus, the amygdala and anterior insula, regions which are important for the identification of emotionally salient information, and the ventral anterior cingulate gyrus and ventromedial regions of the prefrontal cortex, regions, which together with the amygdala and anterior insula appear to be important for the generation of emotional experiences and behaviour in response to this information. Depicted in light blue are regions of the anterior cingulate gyrus and prefrontal cortex, which may have a role in the regulation of emotional behaviour. The arrows (in black) represent the putative functional relationship existing between neural regions important for the three processes. VLPFC, ventrolateral prefrontal cortex; DLFPC, dorsolateral prefrontal cortex; DMPFC, dorsomedial prefrontal cortex; ACG, anterior cingulate gyrus; OBF, orbitofrontal cortex.*

What is the nature of abnormalities in neural systems important for emotion processing in schizophrenia?

Neuropsychological studies

Schizophrenic patients often appear to misinterpret social cues and exhibit poor social skills, with symptoms such as persecutory delusions often emerging as misinterpretations of social interactions and events. Abnormalities in emotional expression identification and emotional behaviour have been demonstrated in patients with schizophrenia in several studies (e.g. Edwards et al[8] and Whittaker et al[9]), and have been associated with the poor social function and dysfunctional emotional experience demonstrated in these patients.[10] The extent to which impaired identification of emotionally salient material is associated with specific abnormalities in the generation and regulation of emotional states and behaviours in patients with schizophrenia remains unexplored.

Neuropathological and structural neuroimaging studies

In schizophrenic patients, these studies have demonstrated abnormal neuronal cell integrity and volume reductions in the amygdala, insula, thalamus and hippocampus (e.g. Wright et al[11]), although there have been inconsistent findings of no reductions in volume within these structures (e.g. Altshuler et al[12] and Chance et al[13]). Regarding regions associated with regulation of emotional behaviour, there have been inconsistent findings regarding the presence of volume reductions within the prefrontal and, more specifically, dorsolateral prefrontal, cortex in schizophrenic patients (e.g. Zuffante et al[14]).

Functional neuroimaging studies

In schizophrenic patients, these studies have demonstrated a failure to activate limbic regions, including the amygdala, in response to arousing and emotive stimuli (e.g. Phillips et al[15] and Crespo-Facorro et al[16]). The finding of absent rather than increased amygdalar activity in schizophrenic patients is somewhat counterintuitive, in view of the predominant persecutory theme of many of the positive symptoms experienced in this patient population. Explanations include increased attenuation of amygdalar responses to overtly threatening stimuli over time because of small structural volumes and identification within these patients of other, more ambiguously threatening stimuli as fearful.[17] Several studies have demonstrated reduced blood flow and reduced activation in regions associated with emotion regulation, including dorsal prefrontal cortex and dorsal anterior cingulate gyrus, in schizophrenic patients (e.g. Andreasen et al[18]).

Summary

Findings from studies of schizophrenic patients have demonstrated in these patients impaired emotion processing, and attenuated responses within neural regions associated with the response to emotive material and regulation of emotional behaviour.

What is the nature of abnormalities in neural systems important for emotion processing in bipolar disorder?

Emotion identification

Many of the symptoms experienced by patients with bipolar disorder, including irritability, distractibility and emotional lability, would appear to be associated with abnormalities in emotion processing, including the experience of emotions of inappropriately high intensity in relation to the context in which they occur, and an inability to regulate mood. In bipolar patients, there have been reports of increased biases towards the identification of stimuli as emotional rather than neutral, and particularly negative, in depressed bipolar patients (e.g. Lyon et al[19] and Murphy et al[20]), and in manic patients, increased negative and positive biases.[19,20] In euthymic bipolar patents, enhanced disgust,[21] and impaired fearful facial expression identification[22] have also been demonstrated. In view of the relatively small number of studies examining emotion processing abnormalities in bipolar patients, it has been difficult to determine whether these abnormalities predominantly represent state or trait effects. Furthermore, the extent to which the abnormal biases towards the identification of emotional material observed in patients with bipolar disorder are associated with the generation of inappropriate emotional states and behaviours, and dysfunctional regulation of these, remains unclear.

Neuropathological and structural neuroimaging studies

In patients with bipolar disorder, these studies have demonstrated reduced glial cell number and density and volume reductions within the ventral anterior cingulate gyrus (specifically, the subgenual region of the ventral anterior cingulate gyrus), and increases in amygdalar volumes, although there are inconsistent findings regarding structural changes within other limbic regions (see Phillips et al[17]). These studies have, however, been unable to distinguish between abnormalities caused by and/or associated with the depressive, euthymic and manic phases of the disorder.

Functional neuroimaging studies

In depressed bipolar patients, compared with healthy volunteers, executive task performance and at-rest studies have demonstrated reduced metabolism in dorsolateral and dorsomedial prefrontal cortical regions, but increased metabolism within the right amygdala. Reduced prefrontal and caudate metabolism to aversive stimulation, and inconsistent findings of decreased,[23] but also increased[24] blood flow in rostral/ventral and subgenual anterior cingulate gyrus have been demonstrated during rest and sad mood induction, respectively. In manic patients compared with healthy volunteers, studies have demonstrated decreases in prefrontal and ventromedial prefrontal (orbitofrontal) cortical activity, and increases in dorsal anterior cingulate gyral and ventral striatal activity, during performance of executive tasks and at rest (e.g. Blumberg et al[25,26] and Rubinzstein et al[27]). There have been conflicting findings regarding basotemporal regions, including the amygdala, in manic patients at rest. No study has examined neural responses to emotional stimuli in these patients (see Phillips et al[17]). Finally, although findings from studies of euthymic patients have demonstrated fewer functional neuroanatomical abnormalities compared with symptomatic patients during executive task performance (e.g. Blumberg et al[25,26]), reports also indicate increased amygdalar and reduced prefrontal cortical activation to facial expressions of fear compared with healthy controls.[22]

Summary

Together, findings from studies of bipolar patients during different phases of illness have indicated biases towards the identificaiton of material as emotive rather than neutral, enhanced activity within regions implicated in the response to emotive material, and reduced activity within regions associated with the regulation of emotional behaviour.

Can schizophrenia and bipolar disorder be distinguished by the pattern of functional neuroanatomical abnormalities during emotion processing?

Findings from studies employing a variety of techniques have highlighted the importance of the amygdala, ventral striatum and other limbic regions, together with ventral prefrontal cortical regions, in the identification and response to emotionally salient information in the environment. In patients with schizophrenia, structural and functional abnormalities in regions important for the appraisal and identification of positive and negative emotional stimuli and production of affective states, including the amygdala and anterior insula, may restrict the range of positive and negative emotions identifiable, a misinterpretation as threatening of non-threatening and ambiguous stimuli, and a decreased range of subsequent affective states and behaviours. Structural and functional abnormalities in the hippocampus and dorsal prefrontal cortical regions, resulting in impairments in reasoning, contextual processing and effortful regulation of affective states, may then perpetuate these abnormalities and symptoms (Figure 22.3).

In patients with bipolar disorder, however, reports indicate enlarged rather than decreased amygdalar volumes, and enhanced rather than reduced activity within the amygdala, subgenual cingulate gyrus and ventral striatum during different phases of illness. Studies have also demonstrated reduced

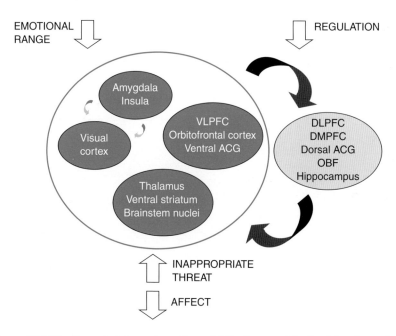

Figure 22.3 *The figure depicts a schematic model for the neural basis of the observed deficits in emotion perception and behaviour in schizophrenia. Structural and functional abnormalities within the ventral system, including the amygdala and anterior insula, may result in a restriction of the range of emotions identifiable, and a misinterpretation as threatening of non-threatening and ambiguous stimuli. These phenomena may be perpetuated by impairments in reasoning, contextual processing and effortful regulation of affective states, resulting from structural and functional abnormalities within the hippocampus and dorsal prefrontal cortical regions. This pattern of abnormalities may be associated with specific symptoms, including emotional flattening, anhedonia and persecutory delusions. For abbreviations see Figure 22.2.*

prefrontal cortical volumes and metabolism in these patients. Together, these findings indicate an 'oversensitive' but dysfunctional neural system for identification of emotional significance and production of affective states, and an impaired system for the effortful regulation of the subsequent emotional behaviour. Specific symptoms of both the depressed and manic phases of illness in bipolar disorder, including prominent mood swings, emotional lability and distractibility may then be associated with these abnormalities in emotion processing (Figure 22.4). To date, however, no information is available regarding the functional neuroanatomy of the switch process to and from euthymia or between mania and depression.

There have to date been relatively few studies examining the specific relationships between abnormalities in the identification of emotional material, the generation of subsequent emotional behaviour, and the regulation of

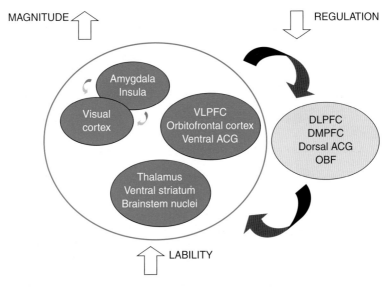

Figure 22.4 *Schematic model for the neural basis of the observed deficits in emotion perception and behaviour, and the relationship between these and the symptoms of bipolar disorder. Enlarged rather than decreased amygdalar volumes, and enhanced rather than reduced activity within the ventral system, suggest a dysfunctional increase in sensitivity of this system to identify emotional significance and produce affective states. Impaired effortful regulation of subsequent emotional behaviours may result from decreases in dorsal prefrontal cortical activity. Specific symptoms of both depressed and manic phases of illness in bipolar disorder, including prominent mood swings, emotional lability and distractibility may be associated with these abnormalities. For abbreviations see Figure 22.2.*

this in either patient population. Further examination is required regarding the nature of the functional neuroanatomical abnormalities associated with different stages of emotion processing in symptomatic and remitted patients, and the effect of medication upon these impairments.

To date, studies suggest that specific abnormalities in the identification of and response to emotional material, and structural and functional abnormalities within many of the neural regions important for these processes, can distinguish patients with schizophrenia from those with bipolar disorder. These findings indicate that increased knowledge of the neurobiology of normal emotion perception will help to further understanding of the complex relationship between specific abnormalities of emotion perception, related deficits in neural systems important for emotion perception, and the symptoms of a wide range of psychiatric disorders.

References

1. Phillips ML, Drevets WC, Rauch SL, Lane RD, The neurobiology of emotion perception. I: The neural basis of normal emotion perception. *Biol Psychiatry* 2003; **54**:504–514.
2. Alexander GE, Crutcher MD, DeLong MR, Basal ganglia-thalamocortical circuits: parallel substrates for motor, oculomotor, 'prefrontal' and 'limbic' functions. *Prog Brain Res* 1990; **85**:119–146.
3. Calder AJ, Lawrence AD, Young AW, Neuropsychology of fear and loathing. *Nat Rev Neurosci* 2001; **2**:352–363.
4. Davis M, Whalen PJ, The amygdala: vigilance and emotion. *Mol Psychiatry* 2001; **6**:13–34.
5. Drevets WC, Neuroimaging studies of mood disorders. *Biol Psychiatry* 2000; **48**:813–829.
6. Damasio AR, Descartes' error and the future of human life. *Scientific Am* 1994; **271**:144.
7. Levesque J, Eugene F, Joanette Y et al, Neural circuitry underlying voluntary suppression of sadness. *Biol Psychiatry* 2003; **53**:502–510.
8. Edwards J, Pattison PE, Jackson HJ, Wales RJ, Facial affect and affective prosody recognition in first-episode schizophrenia. *Schizophr Res* 2001; **48**:235–253.
9. Whittaker JF, Deakin JFW, Tomenson B, Face processing in schizophrenia: defining the deficit. *Psychol Med* 2001; **31**:499–507.
10. Green MF, Kern RS, Robertson MJ, Sergi MJ, Kee KS, Relevance of neurocognitive deficits for functional outcome in schizophrenia. In: Sharma T, Harvey P (eds), *Cognition in Schizophrenia* pp 178–192, Oxford University Press: Oxford, 2000.
11. Wright IC, Rabe-Hesketh S, Woodruff PWR et al, Regional brain structure in schizophrenia: a meta-analysis of volumetric MRI studies. *Am J Psychiatry* 2000; **157**:16–25.
12. Altshuler LL, Bartzokis G, Grieder T et al, An MRI study of temporal lobe structures in men with bipolar disorder or schizophrenia. *Biol Psychiatry* 2000; **48**:147–162.
13. Chance SA, Esiri MM, Crow TJ, Amygdala volume in schizophrenia: post-mortem study and review of magnetic imaging findings. *Br J Psychiatry* 2002; **180**:331–338.

14. Zuffante P, Leonard CM, Kuldau JM, Bauer RM, Doty EG, Bilder RM, Working memory deficits in schizophrenia are not necessarily specific or associated with MRI-based estimates of area 46 volumes. *Psychiatry Res: Neuroimag* 2001; **108**:187–209.

15. Phillips ML, Williams L, Senior C et al, A differential neural response to threatening and non-threatening negative facial expressions in paranoid and non-paranoid schizophrenics. *Psychiatry Res: Neuroimag* 1999; **92**:11–31.

16. Crespo-Facorro B, Paradiso S, Andreasen NC et al, Neural mechanisms of anhedonia in schizophrenia. *JAMA* 2001; **286**:427–435.

17. Phillips ML, Drevets WC, Rauch SL, Lane RD, The neurobiology of emotion perception. II: Implications for major psychiatric disorders. *Biol Psychiatry* 2003; **54**:515–528.

18. Andreasen NC, O' Leary DS, Flaum M et al, Hypofrontality in schizophrenia: distributed dysfunctional circuits in neuroleptic-naive patients. *Lancet* 1997; **349**:1730–1734.

19. Lyon HM, Startup M, Bentall RP, Social cognition and the manic defense: attributions, selective attention, and self-schema in bipolar affective disorder. *J Abnorm Psychol* 1999; **108**:273–282.

20. Murphy FC, Sahakian BJ, Rubinsztein JS et al, Emotional bias and inhibitory control processes in mania and depression. *Psychol Med* 1999; **29**:1307–1321.

21. Harmer CJ, Grayson L, Goodwin GM, Enhanced recognition of disgust in bipolar illness. *Biol Psychiatry* 2002; **51**:298–304.

22. Yurgelun-Todd DA, Gruber SA, Kanayama G et al, fMRI during affect discrimination in bipolar affective disorder. *Bipolar Disord* 2000; **2**:248.

23. Drevets WC, Price JL, Simpson JR et al, Subgenual prefrontal cortex abnormalities in mood disorders. *Nature* 1997; **386**:824–827.

24. Kruger S, Goldapple K, Liotti M, Houle S, Mayberg HS, Cerebral blood flow in bipolar disorder measured with PET: 1. Trait effects at baseline and after mood induction. *Biol Psychiatry* 2001; **49**:87S.

25. Blumberg HP, Eldelberg D, Ricketts S et al, Rostral and orbital prefrontal cortex dysfunction in the manic state of bipolar disorder. *Am J Psychiatry* 1999; **156**:1986–1988.

26. Blumberg HP, Stern E, Ricketts S et al, Increased anterior cingulate and caudate activity in bipolar mania. *Biol Psychiatry* 2000; **48**:1945–1952.

27. Rubinsztein JS, Fletcher PC, Rogers RD et al, Decision-making in mania: a PET study. *Brain* 2001; **124**:2550–2563.

chapter 23

Childhood similarities and differences between schizophrenia and bipolar disorder

Mary Cannon and Kimberlie Dean

Investigation of childhood precursors of adult psychotic illnesses aims to clarify our understanding of aetiologic mechanisms and may ultimately aid the development of stagies for early detection and treatment of the disorder. Reviews of the literature on premorbid characteristics of schizophrenic patients have shown that approximately a third have shown obvious premorbid behavioural abnormalities, including social withdrawal, extreme sensitivity, inability to make friends and poor academic competence.[1–5]

The premorbid functioning of patients who develop affective psychosis has been studied less frequently, perhaps reflecting different views about the aetiology of the condition. Studies comparing the premorbid adjustment of patients with affective psychosis and schizophrenia have found that adjustment is poorer in schizophrenia,[6–9] but without a normal control group could not determine whether the affective psychotic patients were also impaired but to a lesser degree. Prospective and retrospective cohort studies[10–12] have usually, though not inevitably,[13] failed to find significant differences between preaffective psychotic children and normal controls. Poor premorbid functioning is an indicator of poor outcome in affective disorder,[14] and is also a predictor of vulnerability to psychosis in major depressive disorder.[15]

Two studies which have looked at childhood similarities between schizophrenia and bipolar disorder will be described in detail – the Camberwell Collaborative Psychosis Study and the Dunedin Multidisciplinary Health and Development Study.

Camberwell Collaborative Psychosis Study

In this study we used data from a large sample of hospitalized psychotic patients to answer the following questions:

1. Do patients with schizophrenia and bipolar disorder show poor social adjustment in childhood and adolescence compared with controls after adjusting for confounders?
2. If so, how large are the effects and which domains of function are particularly impaired?

Premorbid social adjustment was assessed by maternal recall in patients with schizophrenia (n = 70) and bipolar disorder (n = 28) recruited from a survey of consecutive hospital admissions for psychosis, and in 100 normal catchment area controls.[16]

Our results confirmed the association between poor social functioning in childhood and adult psychosis. The distribution of premorbid social adjustment scores in this sample indicates that social impairment was not confined to a subgroup of patients. All patients showed some degree of social impairment compared with controls. The risk of psychosis was spread throughout the population such that the poorer one's social adjustment, the greater the risk of developing schizophrenia or, to a lesser extent, bipolar disorder. Those with extremely poor social function were at particular risk of developing schizophrenia. Evidence for a linear trend in risk of schizophrenia across population distributions for measures of intelligence quotient (IQ) and behaviour was first shown by Jones et al[17] and has been replicated in a Swedish sample.[18]

Poor premorbid adjustment was not specific to schizophrenic psychosis and was also associated with bipolar disorder. The difference in social functioning among the schizophrenic cases and the bipolar cases was more a question of degree rather than type of abnormality, as found in the British 1946 birth cohort data.[13] The principal difference between bipolar patients and schizophrenic patients was in the area of school adjustment and achievement. Bipolar disorder patients performed as well as controls in school, whereas schizophrenic patients performed badly in this area. The poor school performance of the preschizophrenic children is not surprising in view of previously described intelligence deficits in schizophrenia.[5,18–20] However, adjusting the results for premorbid IQ made little difference, indicating that the preschizophrenic children in this study could meet neither the academic nor the social demands of school. Our results suggested that the school environment, with its emphasis on peer relationships and academic attainment, may be a good arena to detect children who are vulnerable to develop schizophrenia in adulthood, and echo findings from other work.[17,19,21]

Dunedin Multidisciplinary Health and Development Study

Childhood developmental precursors to later schizophreniform disorder and other psychiatric outcomes have been investigated in the Dunedin Multidisciplinary Health and Development Study.[22] This 1-year (1972–73) birth cohort of 1037 children has been assessed six times between ages 3 and 13 years on a range of measures including motor development, language development, IQ, and psychological, social and behavioural adjustment. At age 26, psychiatric status was ascertained using the Diagnostic Interview Schedule and diagnostic criteria for DSM-IV yielded two groups with psychotic illnesses: schizophreniform disorder (n = 36; 3.7%), and mania (n = 20; 2%), and one group with non-psychotic illness: anxiety/depression (n = 278; 28.5%). The Rutter Child scales[23,24] had been administered to the cohort between the ages of 5 and 11 years. Parents and teachers were asked about various externalizing-type problems and internalizing-type problems in the children. Externalizing means antisocial type of behaviour, and internalizing refers more to worries and depression. There was no significant difference between the schizophrenia, mania and anxiety/depression groups on the externalizing or internalizing behaviours. They were all significantly worse than the controls. Parents and teachers were asked to rate two statements regarding each child, 'X is a loner', (a measure of social isolation); and, 'X is not liked by other children', (a measure of peer group rejection). One might have predicted that the social isolation factor would differentially predict later schizophrenia, but in fact those who later developed schizophrenia did not significantly differ from the controls on that measure, whereas the mania group and the anxiety/depression group did. All three groups differed significantly from the controls on the peer rejection measure – again there was no specificity for schizophrenia.

However, neuromotor, language and cognitive developmental impairments in childhood were significantly different from controls only among the schizophreniform disorder group. The relationship between motor, language and cognitive developmental impairment and schizophreniform disorder was independent of effects of sex, socioeconomic status, obstetric complications or maternal factors. These results provide evidence for a pan-developmental childhood impairment that occurs early in childhood and appears to be specific for schizophreniform disorder.

Distribution of developmental impairment among the schizophreniform group within developmental domains

The schizophreniform group was consistently overrepresented (53–56%) in the lowest tertiles (thirds) of the population distribution for motor, language or cognitive development at age 3 years. The summary odds ratios for risk of schizophreniform disorder across tertiles for each of these three developmental measures at age 3 years (Table 23.1) indicated significant linear trends in risk for schizophreniform disorder with increasing developmental impairment within each domain.

Table 23.1 Tertiles of motor, language and cognitive development at age 3 years: percentage of schizophreniform disorder group in each tertile and analysis of linear trends

Developmental domain at age 3 years	Population distribution of developmental scores[a]			Test for linear trend	
	Highest tertile	Middle tertile	Lowest tertile	OR (95% CI)	P value
Motor (% schizophreniform group)	28	16	56	1.6 (1.03 to 2.6)	0.01
Receptive language (% schizophreniform group)	25	22	53	1.6 (1.03 to 2.6)	0.01
IQ (% schizophreniform group)	16	31	53	2.6 (1.3 to 5.3)	0.03

[a] One third of the cohort in each tertile.
IQ, intelligence quotient; OR, odds ratio; CI, confidence intervals.

Distribution of developmental impairment among the schizophreniform disorder group across developmental domains

The risk for schizophreniform disorder with increasing degrees of developmental impairment across developmental domains was examined (Table 23.2). Twenty-eight per cent of the schizophreniform group were in the lowest tertile for all three developmental domains (motor/language/cognitive) at age 3 years, compared with 9.5% of controls (odds ratio (OR) 6.0 (0.9 to 19.1)). A test for linear trend was again significant, indicating a dose–response relationship. Only 16% of the schizophreniform group were not in the lowest tertile at age 3 years for any of the three developmental domains assessed.

Table 23.2 Risk of schizophreniform disorder according to degree of developmental impairment at age 3 years (indexed by being in the lowest tertile for 0, 1, 2 or 3 developmental domains)

No. of developmental domains severely affected (motor/ language/IQ)	Controls (%)	Schizophreniform disorder (%)	OR (95% CI) adjusted for sex and social group
0	42.5	16	Baseline
1	29	31	2.9 (0.99 to 9.01)
2	19	25	3.03 (0.96 to 9.6)
3	9.5	28	6.02 (0.9 to 19.1)
Test for linear trend: OR (95% CI)			1.8 (1.3 to 2.6)
			$Z = 3.6$; $P < 0.001$

For abbreviations see Table 23.1.

Predictive value of developmental deficits in childhood for schizophreniform disorder

The study also examined whether being in the lowest tertile for all three developmental domains (motor, receptive language and cognitive) at age 3 years had any predictive value for schizophreniform disorder (Table 23.3). The sensitivity of this developmental model was 29% (9/31 cases of schizophreniform disorder detected), and the specificity (the proportion of true negatives correctly detected) was 90.5%. The positive predictive value of this 'developmental' model was 14.3% (9/63 subjects), with a false positive rate of 85.7% (54/63 subjects). Addition of information on obstetric complications (low APGAR score, hypoxia-related complication or small for gestational age (SGA)), and maternal rejection to the developmental model resulted in a positive predictive value of 66% (4/6 subjects) but the sensitivity of this 'enhanced' model was only 13% (4/31 cases detected).

Table 23.3 Childhood developmental variables, obstetric variables and maternal variables at age 3 years as predictors of schizophreniform disorder at age 26 years

Risk group	% Sensitivity (n)		% Specificity (n)		% Positive predictive value (n)		% False positive rate (n)	
Developmental risk only	29.0	(9/31)	90.5	(517/571)	14.3	(9/63)	85.7	(54/63)
OC risk only	29.0	(9/31)	90.2	(513/569)	13.8	(9/65)	86.2	(56/65)
Maternal risk only	41.9	(13/31)	80.5	(460/571)	10.5	(13/124)	89.5	(111/124)
Developmental + OC	16.1	(5/31)	95.5	(562/588)	41.7	(5/12)	58.3	(7/12)
Developmental + maternal	19.3	(6/31)	95.7	(555/580)	27.3	(6/22)	72.7	(16/22)
Developmental + OC + maternal	12.9	(4/31)	95.5	(567/594)	66.7	(4/6)	33.3	(2/6)

OC, obstetric complications.

Conclusion

The Dunedin study demonstrates that early-emerging motor, language and cognitive developmental deficits are specific to schizophrenia-spectrum psychiatric outcomes and do not occur in association with other psychotic conditions (such as mania) or non-psychotic psychiatric disorders (such as anxiety and depression). Therefore early developmental impairment is not just a non-specific risk factor for a range of psychiatric pathology in adulthood but provides valuable clues to the processes affected in schizophrenia-related illnesses, although they are a long way from being strong predictors. Emotional problems and poor interpersonal functioning in childhood were associated with a host of different adult psychiatric outcomes at 26 years, including schizophreniform disorder, manic episodes and anxiety/depression disorders. These predictive associations are of actuarial interest – they span more than 15 years and do not exhibit specificity to any one outcome. Lack of specificity is important because it indicates a common pathway to the development of a range of different disorders. Although this constellation of childhood behaviours observed as early as 5 years of age is unlikely to represent a 'prodrome', it is possible that it indexes, more generally, a vulnerable personality that is at risk for all adult psychiatric disorders. One unexpected finding was the lack of a significant association between childhood social isolation (ages 5 to 11 years) and schizophreniform disorders, as this association has been observed in some previous studies of schizophrenia,[1,2,16,17] but it is possible that such peer problems become more evident during adolescence.[25,26]

Rather than thinking about the relationship between childhood problems and later psychiatric disorder in terms of prediction, it may be more helpful to think in terms of trajectories or cascades. Once a child suffers a developmental perturbation in any domain, then its micro- or social environment is changed and the development of brain and mind will also be affected. This might further impinge upon the environment, setting up what has been termed a 'self-perpetuating cascade of abnormal development'.[17] Statistical methods that can encompass dynamic developmental processes rather than merely cross-sectional processes need further development and application. This will not be an endeavour for epidemiology alone. It is increasingly evident that understanding the complex molecular mechanisms underlying brain growth, connectivity and maturation will be crucial to understanding the aetiology of psychosis.

Acknowledgements

Mary Cannon is supported by the Wellcome Trust, the EJLB Foundation and an NARSAD Independent Investigator Award.

References

1. Offord D, Cross L, Behavioural antecedents of adult schizophrenia. *Arch Gen Psychiatry* 1969; **21**:267–283.
2. Rutter M, Psychopathology and development: 1. Childhood antecedents of adult psychiatric disorder. *Aust NZ J Psychiatry* 1984; **18**:225–234.
3. Watt NF, Patterns of childhood social development in adult schizophrenics. *Arch Gen Psychiatry* 1978; **35**:160–165.

4. Hartman E, Milofsky E, Vaillant G, Vulnerability to schizophrenia: prediction of adult schizophrenia using childhood information. *Arch Gen Psychiatry* 1984; **41**:1050–1056.

5. Aylward E, Walker E, Bettes B, Intelligence and schizophrenia: meta-analysis of the research. *Schizophr Bull* 1984; **10**:430–459.

6. Foerster A, Lewis S, Owen M, Murray R, Premorbid adjustment and personality in psychosis: effects of personality and diagnosis. *Br J Psychiatry* 1991; **158**:171–176.

7. Gureje O, Aderibigbe, Olley O, Bamidele RW, Premorbid functioning in schizophrenia: a controlled study of Nigerian patients. *Compr Psychiatry* 1994; **35**:437–440.

8. Dalkin T, Murphy P, Glazebrook C, Medley I, Harrison G, Premorbid personality in first-onset psychosis. *Br J Psychiatry* 1994; **164**:202–207.

9. van Os J, Takei N, Castle D, Wessley S, Der G, Murray RM, Premorbid abnormalities in mania, schizomania, acute schizophrenia and chronic schizophrenia. *Soc Psychiatry Psychiatr Epidemiol* 1995; **30**:274–278.

10. Angst J, Clayton P, Premorbid personality of depressive, bipolar, and schizophrenic patients with special reference to suicidal issues. *Compr Psychiatry* 1986; **27**:511–532.

11. Done DJ, Crow TJ, Johnson EC, Sacker A, Childhood antecedents of schizophrenia and affective illness: social adjustment at ages 7 and 11. *BMJ* 1994; **309**:699–703.

12. Lewine RRJ, Watt NF, Prentky RA, Fryer JH, Childhood social competence in functionally disordered psychiatric patients and in normals. *J Abn Psychology* 1980; **89**:132–138.

13. Van Os J, Jones P, Lewis G, Wadsworth M, Murray R, Developmental precursors of affective illness in a general population cohort. *Arch Gen Psychiatry* 1997; **54**:625–631.

14. Vocisano C, Klein DN, Keefe RSE, Dienst ER, Kincaid MM, Demographics, family history, premorbid functioning, developmental characteristics and course of patients with deteriorated affective disorder. *Am J Psychiatry* 1996; **153**:248–255.

15. Sands JR, Harrow M, Vulnerability to psychosis in unipolar major depression: is premorbid functioning involved? *Am J Psychiatry* 1995; **152**:1009–1015.

16. Cannon M, Jones P, Gilvarry C et al, Premorbid social functioning in schizophrenia and bipolar disorder: similarities and differences. *Am J Psychiatry* 1997; **154**:1544–1550.

17. Jones PB, Rodgers B, Murray RM, Marmot MG, Child developmental risk factors for adult schizophrenia in the British 1946 birth cohort. *Lancet* 1994; **344**:1398–1402.

18. Lewis G, David A, Malmberg A, Allebeck P, Personality and low IQ as possible risk factors for schizophrenia. [Abstract] *Eur Psychiatry* 1996; **11**:242.

19. Jones P, Childhood motor milestones and IQ prior to adult schizophrenia: results from a 43 year old British birth cohort. *Psychiatrica Fennica* 1995; **26**:63–80.

20. Crow TJ, Done DJ, Sacker A, Childhood precursors of psychosis as clues to its evolutionary origin. *Eur Arch Psychiatry Clin Neurosci* 1995; **245**:61–69.

21. Olin SS, John RS, Mednick SA, Assessing the predictive value of teacher reports in a high risk sample for schizophrenia: a ROC analysis. *Schizophr Res* 1995; **16**:53–66.

22. Cannon M, Caspi A, Moffitt TE et al, Evidence for early-childhood, pan-developmental impairment specific to schizophreniform disorder: results from a longitudinal birth cohort. *Arch Gen Psychiatry* 2002; **59**:449–456.

23. Rutter M, Tizard J, Whitmore K, *Education, Health and Behaviour*. Longmans: London, 1970.

24. Elander J, Rutter M, Use and development of the Rutter parents' and teachers' scales. *Int J Methods Psychiatr Res* 1996; **6**:63–78.

25. Malmberg A, Lewis G, David A, Allebeck P, Premorbid adjustment and personality in people with schizophrenia. *Br J Psychiatry* 1988; **172**:308–313.
26. Davidson M, Reichenberg A, Rabinowitz J, Weiser M, Kaplan Z, Mark M, Behavioural and intellectual markers for schizophrenia in apparently healthy male adolescents. *Am J Psychiatry* 1999; **156**:1328–1335.

Index